THE VALUE
OF MEDICINE

THE VALUE OF MEDICINE

Philip Rhodes

M.A., B.Chir.(Cantab.), F.R.C.S.(Eng.), F.R.C.O.G., Dean of the Faculty of Medicine in the University of Adelaide.
Formerly Dean of St Thomas's Hospital Medical School, London, and Professor of Obstetrics and Gynaecology in the University of London

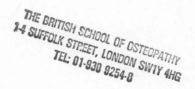
London   George Allen & Unwin Ltd
Ruskin House   Museum Street

F EK

ISBN 0 04 610004 0

Printed in Great Britain
in 11 point Baskerville type
by the Aldine Press, Letchworth

Preface

When I was a House Officer and Registrar, my colleagues and I used to smile indulgently when we saw articles entitled 'Whither Medicine?', written by our elderly mentors. We were sure that we knew what medicine was about. We worked in world-famous hospitals, where excellent work was being done. Our place in the sun was certain and we had to get on with obtaining higher qualifications and increased experience to prove something to ourselves and for the benefit of our future patients.

This was done. A few 'dropped off the ladder' of promotion, but some of us were lucky enough to be climbing nearer to the apex of the pyramid. We were still self-confident and without doubts. After some years as a consultant, or in charge of a university department, one felt reasonably master of the subject of one's choice. There were, of course, still things to be learned, but the clinical surprises became fewer. There was no need to practise one's skills just for the sake of boosting one's ego; they could be used as they were needed for the benefit of the patient. And it was then that the question arose of what exactly was the benefit of the patient. The doubts began to creep in.

Life, and especially human life, is very complex. One scarcely comprehends the ramifications of one's own life, and yet with a brief clinical interview, an examination and a few carefully selected special tests, the doctor is prepared to make a decision about another person's 'benefit'. Of course in many situations, mainly acute, as with agonising abdominal pain, trauma, haemorrhage, the decision is easy. Something must be done, and is. But what about the more difficult areas? With increasing knowledge and experience the doctor comes to have an appreciation of the limitations of therapy. He/she has learned the hard truth that some problems are insoluble. But this appears not always to be known or understood. People like to feel that there must be an answer to everything. It is at this point that you must ask what it is all about.

There is little sense in asking what life is about. It is there in its complexity. But it can reasonably be asked what is the place of medicine in the scheme of things, and what is its value to society. Why is so much effort expended upon it? Are the reasons for it self-evident? Developed countries seem to have expectations of medicine which it cannot always fulfil. And society is ambivalent about medicine too. It may subscribe to humanitarian ideas of medicine and at the same time entertain destructive ideas such as abortion and euthanasia, which destroy life.

Society, and its thinking, have come to have an increasing impact on the aims and objectives of medicine. There was a time when those inside medicine and those outside did not have to question their assumptions, since they were in accord. But now it appears that there is a dichotomy of thought between them. It is the purpose of this book to try to explore it, to find out how it might have arisen. There might even be elements of diagnosis and prognosis on which action could be based. But it is attitudes which determine action and underlying implicit assumptions which determine attitudes.

Underlying, non-explicit assumptions about anything, including medicine, vary both geographically and through time. What is argued here is that assumptions fitting a previous age are being applied to a new situation and so are distorting medicine. My experiences are mainly associated with medicine in Britain and Australia, and it is therefore about these which I mainly write. I have no real experience of medicine in any other cultures. But, at least until recently, even the under-developed countries have pursued a Western-type medicine, adopting its assumptions and trying to apply them to alien cultures. This has often produced unsuitable patterns of health care in those countries. Medicine is not something to be imposed upon a culture from without. It springs directly from indigenous culture and is not separable from it. Cultural diffusion occurs, especially in the adoption of technical changes, but how these are used is shaped by the culture. Moreover, technology is expensive, so how it is used and on what scale is determined by the resources that can be made available. So although British-type medicine and its present development cannot and should not be transposed exactly to fit other cultures, it may well have partial messages for them since it and its ideas are so prevalent, even though its incidence and influence may be diminishing.

The pattern of the book is therefore to explore British medicine through time, that is, a historical method has been used to try to see how thoughts about medicine and its place in society have changed and are changing. This may help to lead to an understanding of the present situation and the way in which present philosophies of medicine do not accord with reality.

The philosophy of medicine has changed over the centuries, as its scope and scale have increased. It is these two, particularly, that have made it change. Its aims and objectives are no longer what they were. It would seem worthwhile, therefore, to try to state them explicitly. The will o' the wisp, the mirage, may then be seen to be what it is and not worth pursuit. The better course might then be chosen.

Adelaide
1975

Contents

Preface   *page* 7

1   *From Magic towards Science*   13

2   *Schism between Religion and Nature, Body and Mind*   25

3   *Charity, Institutionalisation, Materialism*   34

4   *Scientific, Technological and Social Revolution*   42

5   *Mind returns to Medicine*   55

6   *Paradoxes in Medical Thought*   66

7   *Relief and Comfort. Utilitarianism*   75

8   *The Inconsistencies of Medicine and Society*   81

9   *Medical Education*   87

10 *Criticisms of Medical Education*   99

11 *Medicine the Commodity*   112

12 *The Value of Medicine*   118

13 *The Future*   122

14 *Trial Solutions?*   141

Bibliography   159

I

From Magic towards Science

The pathology of bones is written in the fossil record of animals and Man. Tumours and healed fractures and evidence of old inflammation abound. Disease reaches back into prehistory. There has never been a Golden Age without it. Life is a struggle of the living with the environment. There is a ceaseless flux of events in which adjustments of life to the environment are constantly being made. An alteration in one part of the system has repercussions through much of the rest of it. But this is modern thinking, conditioned ever since the publication of *The Origin of Species* in 1859.

The desire to help the sufferer also reaches back into prehistory. There are biological records of animals where the herd will slow its progress to care for and protect its weak and ill members. Some of the herd may show more concern than others for the dis-eased. This seems to be established for elephants, seals and gorillas and may well be true for others too. From anthropological records it can be seen that among the primitive there is often a division of labour in which one or two members of the tribe will be especially turned to when someone is afflicted. There is usually a midwife of sorts, and almost always a medicine-man.

The function of the medicine-man is more to do with magic than with the individual care of the sick, who are usually tended by others with simple nursing care. This is the duty of the family and friends. Only when a disease seems to be especially serious and beyond their scope of simple help is the medicine-man called in. This demonstrates that disease is not seen as being due to natural causes, but that it emanates from the supernatural powers which surround primitive Man. Only equally or more powerful magic can force them to go away and leave the sufferer to recover. The medicine-man understands these powers more than most and has made a special study of them and their capricious ways, and he knows how they may be appeased or driven off. He has magical as well as more mundane knowledge. Both are necessary for his functions, but his credibility and authority reside mostly in his magic. His aura is maintained by his magical practices, incantations, dances, rites, sacrifices, bubbling cauldrons, as well as by his pills and potions. He combines the functions of the priesthood with those of medicine, but the purely medical, in the modern sense, is the lesser part.

Not only is the medicine-man's function to stave off disaster for individuals. He is expected too to protect the tribe from the awful powers which surround it. He must often be the rainmaker and propitiate the tribal gods to prevent the failure of crops and to preserve domesticated animals, and even wild ones too, if the tribe is a hunting one. The mysteries of death, destruction and disease surround the primitive. They are too terrifying to be handled by individuals in isolation. There is an urgent need to institutionalise them. The tribe, as a committee, takes care of the major impending disasters, but appoints a chief executive in the medicine-man to deal with the detail and to be their adviser.

In these apparently simple circumstances may be seen some of the impelling forces of medicine in more civilised societies. In fact, it is probable that the cultural nexus is at least as complicated with the primitive as the civilised. Even now for most people there are struggles with death, disaster and disease, and the responses have become institutionalised, for there is no other way to cope with them. The chief executives of the responses are now qualified medical men and women. There has been a swing away from magic towards medicine as we know it, based more firmly in an understanding of natural causes, but still for many there are lingering vestiges of magic.

The move towards modern medicine, which has entailed changes in the view of the world within which medicine has to function, has been a long, slow process. It is possible to pick out some of the salient features of thought and practice that have changed the face of medicine to what it is today. These features, significant observations, are those which have stepped outside the prevailing philosophy and have shown that it was not sufficient and needed modification. But the acceptance of such modification is slow, and seeps into the particular culture rather than floods it. Indeed, the significance of an advance can only be realised by its relevance to a prevailing world view. All history, especially that of ideas, must be selective, for the historian cannot escape his own time. The position today is taken for granted whilst the signposts from the past which point to the present direction are especially noted. Those pointing in the 'wrong' directions are ignored.

Greek medicine is important, for it is one aspect of a civilisation which has shaped our own in the Western world. It perhaps took over some of the technology of physic and surgery from the Chinese and Indians, who have a long tradition in their use of drugs of various kinds, but they are especially remarkable to us for their use of trephining the skull and Caesarean section. It is probable that the opening of the skull, which was also used by many primitive prehistoric peoples, was an attempt to cure epilepsy and other nervous diseases, as well as for some psychotic states. Incredibly, some patients survived the ordeal, for there is evidence of healing at the edges of the bony wounds in some skulls. Caesarean section may very well have been performed post-mortem, though life in the mother was only recently extinct. Even in Roman times it was thought that mother and baby should be buried separately.

It was the Greeks, especially through Aristotle, who established science and the scientific method of observation, and even to some extent, experiment. Hippocrates took this up and produced the first work of importance in clinical observation. He was the first clinical scientist, though it is possible that the written works known to us were the product of several minds. The titles of the works give some idea of the range – *Prognostic*; *Regimen in Acute Diseases*; *Epidemics*; *Airs, Waters, Places*;

Aphorisms; *Fractures*; *Wounds in the Head.* The importance of trauma at least can be understood, and also the interest in acute diseases, for these always impress themselves upon the observer, and would have done so in Hippocratic times. But what is more remarkable is the relating of disease to race, climate, diet and environment and discussions of prevalence. Also noteworthy is the recognition of the importance of prognosis. Patients may often realise that there is nothing directly that medicine can do for them when they are ill, but they want to know what will happen as a result of their disease. They fear the unknown. If the doctor can make the future known, the illness becomes more bearable.

Hippocrates exemplifies the ability of great men to recognise what can be achieved with the methods available at the time. Then it was eyes, hands, careful observation and recording of what happens when something is done or not done for the patient. The records of Hippocrates still make it possible to recognise malaria, mumps, pneumonia, tuberculosis of the lungs, and demonstrate how to reduce and splint fractures, as well as how to trephine the skull and drain an empyema. But knowledge of anatomy and physiology was elementary. The skeleton, brain, heart, lungs, liver and spleen were known, but apart from some knowledge of the skeleton the theories of function were valueless and misleading. Indeed, the theory that disease was due to some disorder of the four humours – blood, phlegm, yellow bile and black bile – pervaded medicine for almost the next two thousand years.

Hippocrates is now revered for his observation and description, whilst his theory is disregarded. There is a thought here that endears itself to all theorists of the scientific method. It is that if only you will observe and record, without allowing theory to intrude, then good science will result. But theory always does push its way in. It determines what is considered to be worth observation and record, and amid a welter of observations it is theory which determines relevance – what shall be retained and what discarded. There is no science apart from Man as the observer, and experimenter. It is a misleading abstraction to think that science can be entirely objective. It never can be, except at the very simplest levels. Man is always

there, distorting 'external nature' by his presence and inter-
ference and by his isolation of material from nature, for the
purposes of study.

With Hippocrates we see a large injection of common sense
entering medicine. There was a swing away from magic and
theory towards the purely practical function of looking after the
sick. This move away from magic towards soundly based
practice has continued over the centuries, but it is very slow.
As fast as many practitioners try to oust magic, many other
people put it back, in an unreasoning adulation of science and
its achievements.

For many centuries the Hippocratic Oath formed an ethical
basis for medical practice. It is now outmoded in its detail, and
is not subscribed to formally by doctors, as so many of the laity
still think. Its full version, of which there are many variations,
was not written in full until the ninth century AD, though
Hippocrates flourished about the fourth century BC. It is worth
quotation in full here to underline some of the ideas which
infused medical practitioners, both at the time of Hippocrates
and for many centuries after him, and indeed much of its feeling
still imbues medicine today.

'I swear by Apollo the healer, and Asklepios, and Hygeia, and
Panacea and all the gods and goddesses . . . that, according to
my ability and judgment, I will keep this Oath and this stipulation to reckon him who taught me this Art as dear to me as
those who bore me . . . to look upon his offspring as my own
brothers, and to teach them this Art, if they would learn it,
without fee or stipulation. By precept, lecture and all other
modes of instruction, I will impart a knowledge of the Art to
my own sons, and those of my teacher, and to disciples bound
by a stipulation and oath according to the Law of Medicine,
but to none other. I will follow that system or regimen which,
according to my ability and judgment, I consider for the benefit
of my patients, and abstain from whatever is deleterious and
mischievous. I will give no deadly medicine to anyone if asked,
nor suggest any such counsel; nor will I aid a woman to produce
abortion. With purity and holiness I will pass my life and practise my Art. . . . Into whatever houses I enter, I will go there

for the benefit of the sick and will abstain from every act of mischief and corruption; and above all from seduction. . . . Whatever in my professional practice – or even not in connection with it – I see or hear in the lives of men which ought not to be spoken of abroad, I will not divulge, deeming that on such matters we should be silent. While I keep this Oath unviolated, may it be granted to me to enjoy life and the practice of the Art, always respected among men, but should I break or violate this Oath, may the reverse be my lot.' *

The pantheism of Greek medicine is immediately apparent in the Oath, as is the importance of reverence for teachers. It emphasises the brotherhood of medicine and those who practise it. There is the ethical conduct of the doctor towards his patient – not to take life at any stage, and never to divulge secrets. There is a religious appeal about it.

In essence, generations of doctors have lived by the Hippocratic Oath, but the modern world has called and is calling all its precepts into question. It is not now always felt that there should be any special reverence for teachers. They are only doing a job. Teachers themselves may no longer feel the concern for their charges that once seemed necessary. The brotherhood of medicine has been called a closed shop, maintained for the aggrandisement of doctors, and the protection of differentials in monetary rewards. The entry of doctors' sons and daughters into medical schools has been called privilege. Serious concerns of today are medical termination of pregnancy, euthanasia and the confidentiality of patients' records. There is little dedication of doctors to the art of medicine only. They feel that they have their social lives to consider and that medicine should not interfere too seriously with it, and yet they are certain that they should hold a special place in society and be highly rewarded because of it. It is surprising to realise that the tenets of the Hippocratic Oath served as a guide to medical practitioners for over 2,000 years and that now its premises are in large part being discarded.

Greek civilisation and its ideas have continued in their

* This is taken from *Eternal Eve* by Harvey Graham.

rational way to infiltrate the philosophy and culture of the Western world. The early progress of Greek thought was checked by the emotional, religious impact of Christianity. It was not that Christianity was a necessary check, only that institutional-ised Christianity, with its glosses and interpretations of the basic message of Christ, made the cultural environment inimical to the development of the ideas of scientific medicine. Learning became the prerogative of the church; it had a virtual monopoly of teaching and the libraries. In the monastic and clerical life there was no necessary urge to innovate and experiment. Disease was often seen as a visitation of the wrath of God, a punishment for wrong-doing, evil thoughts and sinfulness. Consequently, suffering was seen as justified penance. There need be no fear of death if there is certainty of the life to come. But this comfort is vitiated by belief in purgatory and Hell, whose heavy or light torments depend upon the quality of life lived on earth. So fear of death remained and its terrors were not removed even by ardent belief. God was awful and terrible, and possibly even capricious. It could never quite be known what one's standing in Heaven might be with the unknown admixture of terror, awe, fear, goodness and loving-kindness in the living God.

Yet despite moderating the rate of potential progress of scientific medicine, Christianity gave medicine, and indeed science, jewels of immense value. For science, it put the cer-tainty of order into the universe. A just and jealous God, whose concern is with every falling leaf and minute insect, preserves a regularity in the world and makes it sure that all is not chaos. This certainty is an essential prerequisite for the beginnings of science, for it depends upon the recognition of repeating patterns from which laws and hypotheses may be formulated. If there were no order, there could be no science. If early scientists had not been sure of order there is the possibility that their work would never have begun. Medicine too must partake of this feeling and be grounded in it, but the special role of Christianity in medicine has been its emphasis on the importance of the individual.

Every person is equal in the sight of God. If for no other reason than this everyone has value. The value may not be immediately apparent to someone else, but if the tramp, the vagrant, the fetid, the filthy, the leprous, the diseased, have a special relationship with God, then they must not be scorned. More important is the positive injunction that they must be helped. Although the original religious impetus may now have gone, the spirit is still there. It imbues the better actions of the churches, of communism and socialism. It might even be said that it was the beginning of democracy. There is an outcry when the principle of the importance of the individual is breached, when someone is oppressed. It is not always strong, nor does it always prevail, but it is there. Almost always there is someone to ride to the help of the downtrodden. There is revulsion of feeling over the atrocities of Nazi Germany and of Russia, and feelings of outrage over torture, persecution and violence, wherever they are known.

Although institutionalised Christianity did not provide a good environment for the development of scientific medicine, the institutions of the church did provide care. They looked after the poor, the needy, the distressed and diseased. This was the Christian practical impulse. Those who cared for patients must necessarily have slowly attained a practical expertise. In so doing they were partially denying the creed which suggested that disease was a visitation upon the sufferers for their wickedness. They were interfering in the relationships between Man and God, without explicitly realising it.

Galen's works of the second century AD were those which were accepted by the church for over a thousand years. He has been blamed by some authors for holding back the progress of medicine, but it was not really he who did this, but those who adopted and ossified his work. At least he recognised the need for a knowledge of anatomy, and maybe this was because for part of his career he was a military surgeon. But the church forbade human dissection, so Galen had to be content with dissecting animals. His mistake was to transpose what he learned there to humans, and this perpetuated many errors. He supported the church in his belief that the body was the repository for the soul, a view which prevented deep investigation of the human body, even though his interest in medicine was a partial denial of that doctrine. But it was this attitude which endeared him especially to the clerics, and they elevated his work so much that it became heresy to deny it.

Galen recognised the motor and sensory nerves as well as the sympathetic system, and he knew the effects of section of the spinal cord. But the relationships between breathing and the blood eluded him. He knew that the heart kept the blood in motion, and that there was only blood in the arteries. His predecessors thought that these vessels carried air or 'pneuma', but he believed that the blood ebbed and flowed in the arteries and he never conceived of a circulation.

From Greece, medical and other scientific ideas spread along the shores of the Mediterranean, and for a time Alexandria was the major centre of medical progress until it was carried on to Rome. In the second century AD Soranus, a physician who practised there, described an operation of internal version of the fetus during labour, when there were difficulties in delivery. His place in history is of interest because it shows some early concern for the care of women, though Hippocrates too had shown concern for them. Although there are many isolated instances of an interest in obstetrics and diseases of women shown by medical men, their care resided largely in the hands of other women until about the middle of the eighteenth century. Again, the doctrines of the church are to some extent to blame, for these placed women on an inferior plane and saw them always as a temptation to men. One effect of this was to exclude men from the medical care of women. It has been said that civilisation may be judged by the status and concern given to women, and there is some measure of truth in this. The other interest of Soranus of Ephesus is that he highlights the fact that early progress in medicine could only occur with disorders that were essentially mechanical, such as those of trauma and childbirth. Simple mechanical principles such as those of labour and trauma can usually be easily understood and acted upon.

In the Greek, Alexandrian and Roman eras of medicine, and in those based in Arabia which followed, there were comparatively few medical men, so that care could not be organised in a way which would reach many patients. As so often in the past, medical care was mainly available only to those who could personally afford to pay the doctor. But there were exceptions to this general rule. A hospital was founded in Rome on an island in the Tiber. It was probably first a haven from epidemic pestilence, but later slaves were sent there when they were ill, largely to prevent them being a burden on their masters. And other hospitals were founded, the most famous being at Baghdad, Damascus, Cordova and Cairo. In these sufferers from trauma, eye disorders and fevers were treated, and some of them were used for teaching.

The disintegration of the Roman Empire led to the development of two strands of medicine : the Arabian and the monastic. Judged from our era, Arabian medicine had some scientific successes. The doctors of the time were skilled in some forms of surgery, and in medicine they probably received a fillip from the rise of alchemy. Monastic Christian medicine made very little scientific progress for the reasons previously mentioned. But something was happening in the history of thought, for almost suddenly, about AD 1100, arose the medical school of Salerno. Books, compiling previous knowledge, were written and students were taught. There were even women physicians. Such was the fame of the school that the Emperor Frederick II decreed in 1221 that no one should practise medicine until he had been publicly examined by the masters of Salerno and declared fit to do so.

But the flickering light of scientific medicine and teaching slowly went out at Salerno, to be fanned into life at Montpellier and Bologna, and later at Paris and Padua. There were isolated instances of progress towards our present system of medicine, but their significance can now only be seen in retrospect. They were largely submerged in a welter of what we would now regard as mumbo-jumbo, claptrap, arrant nonsense and supernaturalism. But this rubbish might well have contained jewels for some other culture than our own. The point of view determines the selection from the past. It makes one wonder what is the nonsense of today which is fervently thought to be of importance. Our ideas, highly relevant to us, may be dismissed by the cultures to come.

Suddenly, almost, out of the mediaeval twilight came the brilliance of the Renaissance. Again, this is a concept realised only in retrospect, mainly from the nineteenth century. Those taking part in this rebirth of ideas about the world probably had little idea of what they were involved in. Like us they probably lived from day to day, without recognising the immense forces of social change that were going on about them, and that were destined to alter the shape of the world. They were forging a vessel whose shape they could not foresee and yet which would largely contain the thinking of the Western world. It is likely that we are doing the same, beavering away at small tasks, demonstrating small facts whose inter-relatedness will not be apparent until some later age, and which are already deciding the type of world to come. This is why it is important to lift our eyes to the horizon occasionally, to try to give ourselves a sense of direction. It is now felt that Man should be capable of directing his own destiny, but this cannot be done without some large conception of what has been done and what is likely to be the outcome of trends in thought and culture. For it is thought which determines the sorts of action that are possible. And the results of actions, particularly those which are not foreseen, are often those which modify thinking.

Ideas are like a biological species probing into every corner of the environment, seeking how to exploit weaknesses and gain ascendancy. Or they are like mountain peaks piercing the clouds, which represent the climate of opinion. That climate is nebulous, lacking definition, yet determining our actions as a society. It determines what is said and what is done, what is important and what is not, and what is significant and what is not. It limits the range of what is possible and allowed by that particular culture. A good idea can be stifled by the environment in which it is generated, but if it can grip the imagination of increasing numbers of people, then it is slowly incorporated into the culture, and it will oust conflicting ideas, calling them outmoded. Though some philosophies, like some species, will utterly die out, some will remain in the thoughts of a few, who will nurture them and keep them alive. It is as though an outmoded system of ideas enters a resting phase, waiting to exploit the environment when once more it becomes favourable. This is why history may appear to move in circles, though the movement is more likely in spirals, for historical recurrences are never exactly comparable. The detailed circumstances in which they occur are different. Whitehead puts it well: '. . . a great idea is like a soundless ocean beating on the shores of time in ever increasing waves of specialization'. This means that ideas are buried in the unconscious cultural mind where they motivate individuals to do certain things of whose significance and their own motivation they are often unaware. They are exemplifying in practical detail the implications of the general philosophy of their times.

The actions of individual men and women will normally be contained within the philosophy of their times, but there may be spin-off results of what they do, which do not fit into the perceived system. When these gain sufficient impetus, it is seen that the system will no longer fully contain them, so it must be modified. But although the world view may have changed and actions are modified accordingly, it is often not generally appreciated that the view has changed. It remains unconscious, even though it is a vital determinant of what is done in the future. Medicine has probably reached such a point in the history of ideas. If this is so it is important to find out what those ideas are, and where it is possible they may be leading.

2

Schism between Religion and Nature Body and Mind

The Renaissance may appear as a flood of light suddenly bursting forth, but it in fact lasted from the fourteenth to the sixteenth centuries, three hundred years, and it arose from the previous Middle Ages. The classical ideas of Greece had been held in myriad minds over the earlier millennia and now they gathered strength once more because they caught the imagination in a cultural environment which favoured them, and which was found particularly in northern Italy. It was there that it seemed right to revert to the classical masters, and in so doing the relative dominance of the church and its ideas was partially cast off. Determining factors in this were the existence of the city states of Italy, and the rise of individualism, for the states were small. There were no more than 300,000 people in Florence in 1300, and only 15,000 in Padua. The laity became increasingly influential, especially through the lawyers and the notaries who were combinations of accountant, solicitor and public recorder. They were essential to serve the interests of commerce, industry and finance.

The economic base of society widened because of a steadily rising population, and it was partly this pressure which led to geographical exploration, and to advances in technology and science. The increasing power of business thus challenged the former supremacy of church and state. With shifts in economic relationships came differing social and political values, of which one consequence was the new thinking of science and technology. Until this period it was still believed that everything was composed of the four elements of earth, air, fire and water, and that Man was composed of the four humours of blood, phlegm, yellow bile and black bile.

The invention of printing in Germany in the middle of the fifteenth century was comparable in its effects to the invention of writing itself. Knowledge was no longer confined to manuscripts held in clerical libraries and those belonging to the rich. Books became the potential property of everyone, so that the growth and dissemination of ideas was vastly increased. A revolution in communication occurred. It was added to by literary trends, which moved away from Latin as the vehicle of writing to the vernacular. The world was obviously waiting for printing and for the use of regional language, for both spread rapidly and were avidly adopted.

In science, the year 1543 is often singled out in history because it was then that Copernicus produced his work on astronomy, and Vesalius published *De humani corporis fabrica*. This was the major break with Galen, for Vesalius taught from human dissection. His book was epoch-making, but he was bitterly opposed, especially by the church, for this was at the height of the Inquisition. There were other great anatomists who followed him, such as Eustachius and Falloppius. They again demonstrated the virtue for scientific progress of doing that which is possible at the time. Dissection of animals was well known, but as a technique it had not previously been applied systematically to the human being. There must have been some loosening of the rigidity of thought which held that the body must be inviolate because it was the repository of the immortal soul.

A figure of importance from the sixteenth century was the Frenchman, Ambroise Paré. He was essentially a military surgeon, whose saying, 'I dressed him, but God healed him', has passed into medical history. He was famous as an obstetrician too, and revived the idea of internal version introduced by

Soranus of Ephesus 1,300 years previously. One of the great merits of the Renaissance, of printing and the use of the vernacular was that classical writings in medicine and science became available to a wide audience.

In medicine there was little progress at first, though various diseases were recognised. Diabetes had been known from early times, identified by the sweet taste of the urine. Syphilis became known shortly after the voyage of Columbus to America, and was recognised as contagious. There were, too, the ancient descriptions by Hippocrates of epilepsy and fevers, whilst rashes were commonplace. Thomas Linacre in the early sixteenth century was important because he induced Henry VIII to establish a college of physicians in London, which became the Royal College of Physicians in 1551. This was a recognition of the need to regulate medical practice, and for society to be sure that practitioners had some predetermined knowledge acceptable to their peers. It was also the first attempt to separate the professionals from the amateurs and quacks, with their potentially dangerous nostrums. There may have been an element of self-preservation among the physicians, even one of separatism, but although the college and, later, similar bodies may have been valuable to the medical profession, they have also served as a protection for society. Their foundation has shown that medicine must not be practised in isolation from the needs of society in general, and that its practice is a serious concern of society. This interaction of medicine and society is often an area beset with difficult problems, which are especially apparent at the present time.

Although now they are only of historical interest there were books published in the sixteenth century on children, on childbirth and on diet. They show the areas of interest in medicine at that time. But it was the seventeenth century which brought William Harvey, with his demonstration of the circulation of the blood by a combination of observation, deduction and experiment, which heralds the move towards physiology and to scientifically based medicine. It is perhaps the use of experiment which marks him off from those who had gone before. They had been content with observation, deduction and hypothesis.

Even Harvey, brilliant as he was, was a product of his times.

Genius needs the right environment in which to flourish, and it was this which had changed. The Renaissance and its thought and action had led to the rejection of scholasticism, which was the attempt to reconcile theology and religion with the newer thought which was emerging. It was recognised that there was tension developing between the church's teaching and emergent science and it had been the aim of scholasticism to diminish it and provide an overall view which would contain them both. But there were already those who did not worry overmuch about the effects of their work on theological thought. Galileo had invented the telescope in 1609, and as Basil Willey states it, 'Galileo typifies the direction of modern interests, in this instance, not in refuting St. Thomas, but in taking no notice of him.' This is highly significant. Religion and the church were irrelevant to Galileo's kind of work. He was forced by the Inquisition to accept the teachings of religion, but his researches denied those of the time whatever he felt coerced into saying.

Sir Thomas Browne, that famous literary physician of Norwich, had great difficulties too in reconciling his scientific and religious thoughts. He saw that they often conflicted, and it was because of this that we have his delightful *Religio Medici* (1642–3). His writing suggests that he would have liked religion to win over his mind, but science kept entering in a way that he could not control. He tried to hold both branches of knowledge in his mind at the same time, even when they were irreconcilable. This is an attitude that has persisted ever since. It is fortunate that we do not have to be consistent in all our thinking; perhaps indeed it is impossible to be so, and it would induce neurosis if strict logic ruled our lives, making our assumptions about one subject agree with those in another.

Francis Bacon, especially in his *Advancement of Learning* (1605), saw the dichotomy between science and religion. Religion had made some areas of natural knowledge forbidden, but Bacon tried to escape this by 'arguing that God has revealed himself to man by means of *two* scriptures: first, of course, through the written word, but also, secondly, through his handiwork, the created universe' (Willey). Scientific knowledge was being set free from metaphysical presuppositions. It was being released from having to defer to religion as interpreted by the schoolmen.

William Harvey was in the mainstream of the scientific tradition of the seventeenth century. By 1616 he had shown to his own satisfaction that there was a circulation of the blood, though his *Exercitatio Anatomica De Motu Cordis et Sanguinis in Animalibus* was not published until 1628. He also had more than a passing interest in obstetrics and was among the first to study embryology. The results of his work were published in 1651 in *Exercitationes De Generatione Animalium*. It is worth noting that Harvey was also deeply involved in anatomy and served as a military surgeon of sorts, being with Charles I at the battle of Edgehill in 1642. Like Galileo, and so many others with new ideas, Harvey was severely criticised. The link in the vascular system running from the arteries to the veins was not then known to him, but the invention of the microscope, and its use by Malpighi, the Italian physiologist, demonstrated the existence of the capillaries in 1661. Harvey had died in 1657 so did not know of this vindication of what he had suspected.

There is always a tendency to anatomise history, that is, to cut it up into segments suitable for the purpose of discussion. But, of course, history flows on without overt breaks, and the great men and women of an epoch stand out because they epitomise a group of ideas that are salient and significant for the writer of history. The seventeenth century has seemed to many to demonstrate a watershed, perhaps finally dividing natural science from religion, and making the study of nature a separate discipline. Inquiry, research by observation, experiment and the formulation of hypotheses seemed then to come of age. This was especially shown by the founding of the Royal Society, given a Charter by Charles II in 1663. There were then no separate branches of science. That fragmentation came later. It was then possible for one person to encompass most of what was known, and even make useful contributions to almost any branch of knowledge. In that sense it was a golden age.

These scientific attitudes did not percolate through into medical practice to any marked degree. Only those who could afford it received any real medical attention. However, hospitals, caring institutions, had been founded, notably St Thomas's and St Bartholomew's in London, and they were largely devoted to the care of the indigent sick. But for large numbers of the population there was no medical attention. This lack was not perhaps of much importance, for there was little of specific value to be done for most disorders. There was simple surgery, done without the benefit of anaesthesia, except perhaps that of alcohol or morphia. And there was most elementary obstetrics, but for the vast range of medical diseases there was only general care and nursing, with almost no efficacious drugs. If such should apparently work it was probably as much by suggestion as by their pharmacological effect. Magic here was still as valuable as science. Nevertheless, science was on the move. It might not have been able to accomplish much in therapy but it was beginning to provide the basis for what was to come. This was apparent in the clinical field, too, which was using the old Hippocratic method of observation and record in the hands of Thomas Sydenham, who flourished especially in the third quarter of the seventeenth century.

The investigation of nature had started in Greek times, perhaps because they were uncluttered with emotional reasons for subscribing to a prevalent view of the world, to a cosmology, based on monotheism. It may be that Greek pantheism was liberating. But the institutionalisation of Christianity in the church imposed an authority which was inimical to independent thought about, and investigation of, nature. Renaissance thinking began to change this and reached out ultimately to produce the kind of thought that developed in the seventeenth century, which put religion on a different plane from that of natural science, making them almost irrelevant to each other. This began to put medicine on a different level also, but since Man was still God's creature, medicine was much more conservative than astronomy, geology and other sciences investigating the more obviously physical world, and it retained religious overtones far longer. But despite the commencing separation of medicine and religion the Christian idea of the importance of the individual was there, informing medicine, and giving rise to concern for the ill. Although there were medical practitioners scattered throughout the British Isles, medicine itself was becoming institutionalised in the Royal College of Physicians, and medical care was becoming institutionalised in the founding of some hospitals. Moreover, medical education was obtainable in continental universities, as well as at Oxford and Cambridge, and it was international, many doctors studying at several universities. However, apart from the practical study of anatomy, mainly by demonstration, the education was very theoretical, being based on classical writings, in classical languages, which had comparatively little relevance in the clinical situation. Clinical knowledge was largely gained when the very theoretical doctor went into practice on his own. The best practical study was gained mainly in military or naval service.

Very important in its effects on medicine was the philosophy of René Descartes, whose most famous work was *Discourse on Method* (1637). He has had enormous influence, especially in establishing the theory of dualism, the separateness of body and mind. Much time and energy has been expended in subsequent centuries on getting them back together again, with philosophers swaying back and forth between idealism and materialism. As with religion, science has tended to find these disputations irrelevant. Without positively asserting that it did so, science has adhered to materialism – a belief in a world 'out there', separate from the observer, which could be investigated. It has led to great advances in understanding the physical world in physics, chemistry and astronomy, but may well have held back biology and medicine, because it ignored the elements of mind, behaviour and time. Whitehead has described it as the doctrine of 'simple location', that is, that a piece of matter is 'here' in space and 'now' in time. Despite its success in investigation and in technology it is a notion of high abstraction from the real situation. It allows for a description of the world in measurable and mathematical terms, whilst leaving out of account so much that is of importance in human life. Its very success has been distorting. One aspect of this is that the doctrine excluded psychology, psychiatry, sociology and behaviour from legitimate study. These have had to creep back into science in a roundabout fashion through philosophy, rather than through natural science. The adherence to underlying assumptions, epitomised in different philosophies, explains why even today natural scientists still have difficulty in accepting these new disciplines of psychology and sociology as other than soft options to the rigours of science. Some of them define science narrowly, almost in seventeenth-century terms.

The emancipation of science from the yoke of religion freed the genius of Newton. He published his *Principia Mathematica* in 1687. His scientific explorations were a marvellous vindication of the methods of the new natural science. He established laws of nature with regard to motion and gravity. Not only did these describe what happened in certain situations; they also, by their generality, forecast what would happen and 'explained' it. He brought order into astronomy and physics. He was a great unifier. It was in this that his brilliance resided. Although Newton embraced religion and believed that his work supported the church's teaching in showing nature as the creation of God, it was the detachment of nature from God which was the prerequisite for his investigations. Whatever his own presuppositions may have been, the framework within which he operated belied him. Certainly this is how he is interpreted now.

A usual view of scientific method is that the scientist forms a hypothesis, patiently gathers facts, so confirming or denying his hypothesis. If the facts fit the hypothesis, then it is accepted. If they do not, then the hypothesis is discarded or amended. This is the apotheosis of Materialism, which separates the observer from the observed. It totally ignores the possibility that observing and experimenting may influence the observed in unsuspected ways, and it ignores the fact that any experiment, with its control of as many factors as possible in what is observed, has abstracted greatly from the real situation. Moreover, the hypothesis has to be framed on a basis of underlying assumptions, most of which are implicit and not consciously realised or recognised. The conditions of experiment and observation postulate a world view which is not explicit, and which is dependent upon the prevailing climate of opinion, which is the inherited cultural tradition. It pervades any study. The sorts of facts to be gathered together are predetermined by this unspoken philosophy of the scientist, and importantly it is this which allows of the decision as to which facts shall be excluded from consideration. But the patient gathering of facts has its value, for when they have reached a certain critical mass they form the basis on which some genius may speculate and alter the view of the world and its works. In science there is room for the grand speculation as well as for the fact-gathering. For most of us it is the grand unifying speculation that has the greatest significance. It is what Newton did for matter with his laws of motion and gravity. Since his time there have been Darwin, Freud and Einstein with their similar glimpses of grand design which have changed human direction.

3

Charity
Institutionalisation
Materialism

Newton's success in his investigations of the material world affected the growth of science and of medicine in the eighteenth century. There was no great liberation of thought such as had occurred during the Renaissance and up to the seventeenth century. In this way the eighteenth century was quieter. It was a time of steady progress in many fields. It was ushered in by what was called the Augustan Age in literature, progressed into Dr Johnson's England and closed with the Romantic poets. There was a spirit of optimism, Steele among others advocating cheerfulness.

The mainstreams of medicine and of science ran parallel rather than convergently. Indeed, it was not until well into the twentieth century that the physical sciences and medicine really came together to make an impact in an era of high technology. Looking back on the eighteenth century it seems to have been a time of fact-gathering after the grand speculation generated by Descartes and Newton. It was to some extent a time of invention of new techniques of investigation of the world, and of the application of technology. Both the Industrial and Agricultural Revolutions had their origins towards the end of the eighteenth century, and they were practical triumphs of the new scientific thought.

Although there were few notable evidences of new thinking in medicine, the social changes of the eighteenth century were important in that they ultimately shaped the form in which medicine was to progress. Some consideration of the shifts in society is therefore worthwhile. Cultural attitudes to medicine, and within society, were in more of a transition phase than they always are. Crystallisation of ideas was beginning to emerge from the relatively amorphous mass, even though those ideas were not yet converging from their separate disciplines. Disparate development in religion, philosophy, society, science, technology and medicine seems characteristic of the age, yet all were forming the backcloth against which medicine functioned in the succeeding centuries.

The major influence on medicine in this hundred years came from the charitable impulse. There had always been some isolated concern for the poor, sick and needy, but it was in this period that there came the beginnings of organisation to help them. The fillip came largely through John Wesley and the foundation of Methodism, which was a most powerful social force at the time. Its effects continue now through socialism in many of its forms and through the trade unions. The background of this social progress was increased economic prosperity and a rising population. Both affected each other. The economic improvement was partially channelled into social improvement, which raised the birth rate, which in its turn provided the labour to expand the economy. The population of England and Wales in 1701 was about $5\frac{1}{2}$ million, of which about 670,000 were in London. There were few other towns of any size. By 1801, after the first census, the population was 9 million.

The philosophers struggled with their various themes. They inherited Locke from the end of the seventeenth century. He had published his *Essay Concerning Human Understanding* in 1690. The torch passed to Berkeley and Hume, but they had little influence on the movements in science and medicine in philosophical attempts at reconciliation of the conflicting ideas of their time. Berkeley was perhaps the most famous of idealists, so reacting to the materialism firmly established by Newton's experiments. However, Newton was a theist and firmly believed that what he demonstrated in the physical world showed God's works and glorified Him. As Willey remarks, 'The Universe had been explained, and – what gave added zest to their satisfaction – explained by an Englishman – and a pious Englishman at that'.

The problems of body and mind, set asunder by Descartes, exercised few in medicine. Most doctors appear to have taken a Materialist position, even though they may not have professed it overtly. But there was difficulty in explaining life entirely in terms of physical matter. Stahl, Professor of Medicine at Halle, introduced the idea that the soul impelled the body through 'anima', a kind of vital spirit. The obvious inter-relations of body and mind caused the rise of animism and vitalism, the latter postulating a vital principle imbuing all life. They were aberrations in the general movement of science and medicine, for they explained nothing and only substituted one name for another, so compounding a difficulty.

In science, Fahrenheit introduced the mercury thermometer in 1714, having produced an alcohol thermometer a few years earlier. The Reverend Stephen Hales investigated plants, and was the first to measure the blood pressure directly by inserting a tube into the carotid artery of a horse. He paved the way for Priestley to discover oxygen by showing how to collect gases, having studied water evaporation in plants. Priestley found oxygen in 1774, but did not fully appreciate the significance of his finding. He told the Frenchman, Lavoisier, about it over dinner. Lavoisier then continued the work and exploded the phlogiston theory for all time. This had suggested that all matter consisted of some basis together with phlogiston, which escaped into the air when the substance was burned. But, in fact, on burning, many substances increase in weight by oxidation, whereas if phlogiston escaped from them they should lose weight. As a result of this work the significance of respiration became a little clearer, and one offshoot of it was to generate interest in ventilating buildings.

Technology flourished, ushering in the Industrial Revolution, traditionally said to begin about 1760. In 1769 came Watt's steam engine and Arkwright's water frame, and the following year Hargreaves perfected his spinning jenny. The factories were now firmly established, and people were increasingly attracted to the towns and cities, hoping for employment. They swelled the numbers of the urban populations and reproduced too easily in inadequate slums where disease and death were rife. At about this time Goldsmith wrote his poignant poem 'The Deserted Village' (1769), deploring the drift from the countryside, but this was not to be halted.

Crompton's mule, an improved machine for spinning yarn, was invented in 1779 and fed the growth of the textile mills, whilst in 1781 Boulton and Watt perfected a steam engine with a rotary motion. Manufacturing changed from being a cottage industry and needed armies of people gathered together in one place. Towns and cities grew. Such was the demand for labour that children toiled in the factories and mines as well as men and women.

The Agricultural Revolution began a few years before the conventional beginning of the Industrial Revolution. The century had seen increasing enclosures of land, which changed the base of rural society. More intensive farming was begun, notably by Coke of Norfolk and Bakewell of Leicester, to increase yields of crops and animals when there was a diminished labour force. They were responding to the drift to the towns.

Scientific medicine went on its way. Deventer produced a book on obstetrics in 1701. The great Dutchman, Boerhaave, flourished in the first few years of the century and, like so many others of this century, he was renowned for his clinical acumen. He was also a great teacher at Leyden, a university which remained in the forefront of medical education. In 1721 Lady Mary Wortley Montagu came back from the East with stories of vaccination against smallpox and paved the way for Jenner in 1796 – another example of how slowly new advances are taken up – to perform his first vaccination using cowpox.

Surgery was in the hands of men like Cheselden of St Thomas's, who published his *Osteographia* in 1733 and it remained a standard work for many years. As its name implies it was about bones and was essentially anatomical with some allusions to pathology. But it demonstrates that medical education was mainly theoretical at first, being a study of anatomy and botany and chemistry, until clinical work was studied as an apprentice in the now burgeoning hospitals. Other surgeons of the century were Douglas, who described the peritoneal pouch in the pelvis; Pott, who described his fracture near the ankle, and Heberden, who described the bony nodules of osteoarthritis. They were practical men.

Apart from Boerhaave, clinical medicine was practised in its highest form by men such as Richard Mead, among many others. Therapeutics was still unscientific by our standards, but William Withering described the actions of extract of foxglove on the heart in 1785, and this led to the discovery of digitalis. But there were few drugs of potent action, except the time-honoured opium derivatives, though Dover introduced his pain-relieving powder in 1732. In 1753 James Lind found that limes prevented scurvy in sailors, an interesting fore-runner of preventive medicine. This made long sea voyages less hazardous, for scurvy is debilitating and subscorbutic states were a cause of ill-temper, and even mutiny. Cook's voyages, discovering Australia (1770 and after), were in part made possible by this discovery. Experimental medicine was pursued especially by John Hunter, whose questioning mind took him in several different directions, in exploring growth and in infectious disease, particularly venereal, with which he deliberately inoculated himself to investigate its natural history. In so doing he was able to distinguish gonorrhoea and syphilis, but died as a result.

It was a time of great advance in midwifery. Naboth described the follicles of the cervix; there was an English edition of Deventer's book *The Art of Midwifery Improved*; William Hunter was one of the best practitioners; the obstetric forceps was introduced and their use was codified and made relatively safe by the master of British midwifery, William Smellie; Fielding Ould was in Dublin and advocated episiotomy, the incision in the perineum to facilitate birth, whilst Harvie in London wrote on the method of delivery of the placenta, and there were several others such as Levret in France, Pugh and Manningham, and their manifold writings show that this was a heyday in obstetrics. Moreover, it shows an increasing concern with women, and socially this was also seen in the fact that many of them were now being educated in schools, and novels were being written mainly for them. The cult of such writing began with Samuel Richardson, whose heroines were Pamela, and Clarissa Harlowe. In 1792 Mary Wollstonecraft wrote her *Vindication of the Rights of Woman*, and Jane Austen and Fanny Burney flourished towards the end of the century.

The activity in midwifery contributed to the rising population and this began to cause some anxiety, as manifested in *The Essay on the Principle of Population* by Malthus (1798). The large numbers of people in the towns and cities caused much poverty, about which Eden wrote in *The State of the Poor* in 1797. The vast numbers of these poor men, women and children stirred the charitable impulse, and this probably gained emotional and religious fervour from the preaching activities of John Wesley, and the founding of Methodism. It was an uncomfortable religion in many ways, which whilst carrying the divine message also managed to contain a puritanical streak in renouncing what are now thought to be some of the innocent pleasures of the world. This same meanness and vindictiveness is still to be seen in its offshoots in socialism and the labour movement. Those not fully subscribing to their aims and methods are outside the charmed circle and can therefore be castigated and vilified. Perhaps all fervent social movements have some compounding of good with unpleasantness, and may take much time in the development of tolerance.

The social movements were many in bettering the lot of the people. They include street lighting, education for boys and girls and the founding of hospitals and other charitable institutions. Lighting was introduced into Westminster in 1734, and it was brought about by a group of residents, who managed to arrange that householders should pay for it. It increased the security of the city, and showed what might be done by a band of enthusiasts without general public support. The rash of hospital building was very remarkable as shown by this list:

1719 Westminster Hospital
1725 Guy's Hospital
1733 St George's Hospital
1739 Queen Charlotte's (Maternity) Hospital

1740 London Hospital
1745 The Middlesex Hospital
1745 The Foundling Hospital
1747 Lying-in Wards at the Middlesex Hospital
1750 City of London Maternity Hospital
1765 New Westminster Lying-in Hospital
1784 Lying-in Hospital in Edinburgh
1784 Lying-in Hospital in Vienna
1790 St Mary's Hospital, Manchester
1793 The Retreat, York Maternity Hospital, Edinburgh
1796 Royal Sea Bathing Hospital, Margate

The founding of these hospitals shows a variety of motives. There must have been a felt need for them compounded of a realisation of the enormities of poverty and disease in a commencing industrial, urbanising era, the charitable impulse, the technological advances in midwifery, the numbers of injured sailors and soldiers as a consequence of the wars, and of a rising rich class with money to spare for charity, and the time to dispense it. Political changes too helped for there was discontent with parliamentary representation, which matched, in its calmer British way, the French Revolution which started in 1789. Social changes only rarely come singly. The general impulse for change has many specific exemplifications.

Further evidences of concern for the human condition are seen in the founding of the Royal Humane Society in 1777 and the passing of an Act in 1788 to regulate the employment of small children as chimney-sweeps. It was an age of institutionalising social activities. There had previously been many isolated private enterprise attempts to do this, but this was the time when it gathered strength. In this time can be seen other examples of banding together, for the Royal Academy was founded in 1768 by Joshua Reynolds, and scientists started a *Journal of Natural Philosophy, Chemistry and Other Arts* in 1797, and founded the Royal Institution in 1800. Trade unions were just beginning, and the reaction to them was seen in a regulating Act directed towards containing them in the Combination Act of 1800. Even the navy was not exempt from these social changes, for there were mutinies at Spithead and the Nore in 1797, showing a special impulse for the aggrieved to rise against their oppressors.

Physical science became more emancipated and looked less over its shoulder to see what effects it might be having on the church and its doctrines. Medicine pursued a parallel course, taking comparatively little notice of the other sciences. It was collecting its own clinical scientific facts, and very much improving its technology in midwifery. The scientists and the doctors were coming together, but the major impact of social change was seen at first more in medicine than in science. Here the rising status of women allied with obstetric advance led to the institutionalising of midwifery, whilst the rising tide of population in London, the maimed serving men and a belief in the improvements in medicine and surgery, even if they were in part illusory, institutionalised those disciplines also. There was an unexpressed feeling abroad that society must take care of its more unfortunate sufferers. It was realised that what had been done in the past on an entrepreneurial basis was now no longer enough. By organisation of midwifery, surgery and medicine into institutions the technological benefits of these disciplines could be brought within the range of a greater number of people. It was a system which paved the way and prepared for the achievements in science and medicine of the nineteenth century. The two began to come together.

Medicine was still practised in the eighteenth century against a philosophical background of Newtonian physics. The patient was very like a lump of matter without antecedents and without potential. He was here and now, and treated in isolation from his surroundings, just as scientists thought they could investigate matter. The unacknowledged code of materialism reigned in the practice of medicine.

4

Scientific Technological and Social Revolution

The nineteenth century was one of remarkable progress. The Victorians were aware of it themselves. They felt it was in the air and inevitable. The eighteenth century had shown them the way. Materialism had been vindicated by its scientific and technological successes. There is a link between the sentiment of inevitable progress and *laissez-faire* economics, which dominated so much of the era. There was a certain rectitude about the British way of life and British institutions. The whole period demonstrates the inter-relatedness of progress in several fields at once. New ideas caught on quickly and were put into action, because the climate of opinion was ripe for doing so. Not only were people receptive to new ideas, but there was the prosperity and financial backing to translate them into action. Scientific, medical and technological progress require, it seems, a suitable background of receptive thought in the educated populace and a thriving industry and commerce, from which to derive nourishment, both in ideas and in money. The Middle Ages deprived science and medicine of important mental and physical support. The nineteenth century gave them both unstintingly.

America and France had been convulsed on the one hand by the War of Independence and on the other by the Revolution.

The War ended in 1783, and the Revolution stretched from 1789 to Waterloo in 1815. They and the American Civil War of 1861 to 1865 were indicative of social and political change. Britain, after Waterloo, was not directly involved yet absorbed some of the democratic revolutionary feeling from both. Her social upheaval was carried through largely without bloodshed because of her economic and parliamentary stability. These were not absolute and there was discontent under the surface, but the organs of the establishment could adapt to the social forces by small degrees. When ground is ceded by the privileged there is no need for bloody revolution.

Economic strength was built on the technology of machines, the mines and iron ore as well as agriculture. There was a large market both within and outside the country. The demands for labour were met by the rising population, of about 13 million in 1815, increasing to 26 million by 1871. People may have worked in dark satanic mills and lived in filthy hovels, but the death rate diminished, the birth rate rose and there was an influx of immigrants particularly from Ireland. Perhaps medical progress and care made some slight contribution to better health but their benefits were thinly spread. Public health measures too might have been involved, but in the early years of the century they were rudimentary. The rising population was due to teeming life battering away at its inhumane environment, and making a success of it, as a species, though at great cost to individuals.

Britain obtained an edge on the rest of the world by her freedom from war and revolution, which gave her an early start in science and technology. By 1870 her foreign trade was four times that of France, Germany and Italy put together. As a result, London became the centre of the world's banking and commerce, and perhaps one of the most significant exports was her emigrants. They moved to the colonies in millions, and the results of that mass migration are still being worked out, for the people went to America, Canada, Australia and New Zealand, carrying their cultural values with them, and maintaining ties of all kinds with the mother country.

The aristocrats were gradually ousted from their pre-eminent position by the entrepreneurs of industry, commerce and

banking. Royal supremacy had previously been brought under
control by the aristocracy and it was more or less ended by the
times of the Regency, for a constitutional monarchy to be
established under Victoria. The power passed to the new rich,
who made enormous amounts of money and became landed
gentry, often expressing a philistinism in their buildings,
furniture, decoration and art which is still often regrettable,
even though there has been renewed interest in the cultural
objects of the Victorian Age.

This new peak of society did not, in historical terms, remain
for long. Its wealth depended too much on a poor exploited
substratum, which gradually gained strength during the period.
It was of course aided and abetted as a movement by many of
the ruling class, which contained elements of philanthropy. By
1808 the activities of Wilberforce, the Clapham Sect and
Charles James Fox had finally banished slavery from the
British Empire. The antagonism of working-class people to the
manufacturers' machines, which some of them saw as depriving
them of a living, issued in the Luddite Riots of 1811 when
machines were smashed. The mobs of London, and those of
other cities where manufacturing sucked in the population from
the rural areas, caused alarm, which was answered by the
setting up of Commissioners of Police in the Metropolis in
1811, though Sir Robert Peel's famous force did not actually
come into operation until 1829. Meanwhile Peterloo had
occurred. The army had been called out to a potentially
militant working-class meeting near Manchester and in the
scuffles eleven people died. It became known as the massacre
of Peterloo. The repeal of the Combination Act in 1824 made
trade unions legal, and in 1829 a Relief Act was passed, removing some of the disabilities under which Roman Catholics
suffered. In 1831 King's College, London, was founded and
students were admitted there without reference to their creed.
Formerly, the older universities had allowed admission only to
Anglicans.

The Tolpuddle martyrs had tried to found an agricultural
trade union, and under a technicality three were hanged and
400 transported. That was in 1834, and two years later the
London Working Men's Association was formed, and two years

after that the People's Charter Movement began. It was essentially for political reform but it demonstrates with the other examples the ideas of the time, with the ordinary people struggling for a place in the sun. A further social movement was the Co-operative Society beginning in 1844, and by 1869 the Trades Union Congress was set up, and two years later a Trade Union Act was passed. It was amended again in 1876. By 1884 it was recognised that property should not be the only criterion for the exercise of a vote for a member of parliament, and in that year a Franchise Act was passed. In 1872 the ballot box had become secret for the first time. The nineteenth century saw a quick building up of pressure groups of all kinds. Those in the political sphere only demonstrated overtly the groundswell from which they sprang.

The plight of women and children in the mines and factories was often appalling. Lord Shaftesbury saw the need for their protection and introduced a series of Factory Acts, which mitigated some of the worst perpetrations upon these weaker members of society. John Stuart Mill campaigned for women when he was a member of parliament, saying that they should have equal rights with men in voting. The movements designed to obtain rights for the individual were gathering strength during this century. But naturally there was some opposition, as shown in much repressive and often cruel legislation. Since materialism had such a hold, and economic progress seemed so secure, *laissez-faire* must have appeared to be right. And each man was thought to have the capability of raising himself through society by his own exertions. The best poor were those who did not ask for charity, but struggled to keep their homes clean, patching their clothes and pulling in their belts. It is no surprise that one of the books with the greatest circulation was Samuel Smiles' *Self Help* published in 1859. But even this idea was not fully believed for there was a Poor Law Amendment Act in 1834, which improved the bases for helping the poor. In 1888 the Local Government Act came into force, and this shows the increasing institutionalisation needed for social action to occur. The local governments became responsible for looking after the poor.

Children were not forgotten. The Society for the Prevention

of Cruelty to Children started in 1884, and increasing provision was made for their education. The population became increasingly literate, as ideas began to flow more easily because transport had improved with the building of railways and roads, and telegraphy had been handed over to the Post Office in 1869. Towards the end of the century, the popular newspapers had begun, a development only possible when there was a fair degree of literacy.

It was a time of improvement in public health. In 1838 Edwin Chadwick had arranged for a group of doctors to look into destitution and death in cities. They found deficiencies in water supply, sewerage and rubbish disposal. A cholera epidemic struck the metropolis in 1848, so reinforcing their findings. The government response was to set up a Central Board of Health Commissioners, but a further cholera outbreak in 1865 led to legislation laying upon local authorities the duty to appoint sanitary inspectors and make arrangements for a pure water supply, adequate sewerage and waste disposal.

Local authorities were not always very strong in the early nineteenth century, but a Local Government Act of 1888 gave them reasonable powers, leading the way to their present functions in many areas of public concern. The London County Council began in the year of the Act. There is to be seen in this the usual form of social progress. A few people entertain ideas about alternative ways of doing things. They see that a present method may be improved. Some of them get together to put their new ideas on a factual basis so that doubters may be convinced of the strength of the case for change from accepted ways. Little progress is made at first, but then the problem crops up again. It is increasingly realised that the previous solutions were not very good. Government then steps in, either at local or central level, and starts a board or committee, which then has to hire officers to do the work for them executively. It is a time-worn system, with unfortunate inbuilt delays. In this instance Chadwick saw the problems of urbanisation, as did many others, probably long before 1838, but could see no way of doing anything about them. His advisers, in broad terms only, showed him the probable diagnosis. To obtain further concrete evidence and to get things done needed governmental resources. The problems could not be dealt with centrally so they were handed on to local authorities. They too could not function as they should have, so they in their turn had to be strengthened. In restrospect this was quite a quick process of social movement, but it took at least fifty years, and even then the problems first analysed were not all solved practically and quickly everywhere in the realm. A further phase in this developmental process was seen when the Health Board of 1865 evolved into the Ministry of Health in 1919.

It is against the background so far sketched that scientific and medical progress must be seen. And just as social progress takes time, so does the acceptance of innovations and discoveries in science and medicine. They can only be entertained as interesting at first. Later their relevance to the practical world can be understood, but that requires adjustment of thinking on the part of a critical mass of people. When this has reached the required number, whatever that might be, the technology for introducing the discovery for the benefit of large numbers is developed. Thought precedes discovery, and evidence has to be obtained to persuade others who are not easily convinced that a discovery is valid. Then ever-increasing numbers have to see its relevance, fit it into their own field and background of knowledge, and give it financial and moral support. Only then can something be done about it.

Anatomical investigations continued. Rosenmüller described the remnants of the mesonephros in the broad ligament of the uterus; von Baer saw the dog's ovum; Cloquet described the anatomy of hernia; Carus demonstrated the curve of the birth canal; Gaertner described his duct; all these were in the first fifty years of the century. Anatomical teaching continued on its steady way, and became the foundation of scientific medicine.

The science of physiology also first began in this century. There had been many physiological discoveries prior to this, notably by John Hunter, but the nineteenth century was the time of separation of anatomy from physiology. The distinction of physiology owed much to Sir Charles Bell, the anatomist, who demonstrated that the dorsal roots of spinal nerves conveyed sensation, whilst the anterior roots were motor, and further physiological themes were developed by Müller, Helmholtz, Hertz, Waller and Ludwig. Müller, among other things, was the namer of the Müllerian ducts; Heimholtz investigated the mechanisms of the eye, and in his work with Hertz introduced electro-dynamics into the study of living tissues. Waller discovered Wallerian degeneration in severed peripheral nerves and Ludwig concentrated much on blood pressure and renal function. Pupils under Müller were Henle the anatomist, especially now known for the histological loop in the kidney, and Virchow who founded cellular pathology.

By 1804 Dalton had established the Atomic Theory in chemistry. Humphry Davy had written on agricultural chemistry in 1813, and two years later chemical equations had been evolved. This was because chemical elements were being defined, for Davy in 1806 had described sodium, potassium and magnesium, as well as chlorine.

In medicine Auenbrugger showed the value of percussion in 1761, but it was not introduced on any scale until it was popularised by the Frenchman, Corvisart, about 1808. He also did much work on the heart and showed the difference between dilatation and hypertrophy. In 1817 Laënnec produced his first stethoscope and published an account of the instrument two years later. Auscultation was picked up by Lejumeau in 1822 and he used it for listening to the fetal heart. In 1827 Bright wrote on renal disease from Guy's Hospital, and in 1843 Lever, of the same hospital, showed albuminuria in eclamptic women.

Surgery took steps forward. Ephraim McDowell of Kentucky performed a successful abdominal ovariotomy in 1809. In 1817 came the first successful operation for an abdominal pregnancy by John King. In 1831 Syme published his *Principles of Surgery*. Two years later, one of his colleagues, Liston, was appointed Professor of Surgery at University College Hospital, London. It was in 1846 that Joseph Lister watched Liston perform an amputation at that hospital under ether anaesthesia. In 1840 Mettauer of Boston successfully repaired a vesico-vaginal fistula.

The first real stirrings of anxiety about pain and sepsis in surgery began. Laughing gas was used in dentistry by Wells in

1844, and ether was used for the first time in the United Kingdom in 1846 at Liston's operation mentioned above. Simpson first experimented with chloroform in 1847 and it was used at a confinement of Queen Victoria's in 1853. Semmelweiss wrote on puerperal sepsis, and Oliver Wendell Holmes had a flash of insight in 1843 when he recommended that the hands should be washed in chloride of lime before operations.

These various lines of progress all continued into the second half of the nineteenth century, and such was the pace of discovery that it is hard to try to pick out the strands of advance to the present day. The names of the great of those days are still eponymously attached to a large number of medical disorders, structures and symptoms. Accounts of medical history leave out of account the innumerable first-class practitioners and teachers, whose contribution to the ethos of medicine and to its spreading far and wide is incalculable.

The institutions of medicine increased enormously. Hospitals especially grew up in many areas of the country where there had formerly been only a rudimentary service, provided usually only by a few single-handed practitioners. These were often remarkable men who would turn their hands to any medical problem as well as being guides, mentors and friends to their patients. But the nineteenth century saw the seeds sown for their eclipse as medicine, surgery and midwifery became increasingly specialised under the impact of fresh discoveries. After this time it was no longer possible for every doctor to encompass all there was worth knowing to help him in the care of the sick. By 1900 there was specialisation in metabolism, cardiology, paediatrics, neurology, ophthalmology, oto-rhino-laryngology and dermatology. Journals of various societies and specialties began to appear in profusion. Although there had been a Company of Barber-Surgeons since 1540, the Royal College of Surgeons did not properly start until 1800. A Midwives Institute began in 1881.

Sketchy though this brief look at history has been it is no longer possible nor desirable to pick out details. The survey has shown some of the elements which form attitudes to medicine. They are magic, science, Christianity (or other religions in other countries), charity, political and social movements, commerce, industry, war and institutionalisation. There has been some demonstration that medicine depends on all these for its practice, and that discoveries and innovations in science and medical science and the delivery of medical care need a favourable climate of opinion and a development of technology for their application. Up to this point in history, i.e. of the nineteenth century, the technology often had to wait on physical discoveries in other sciences, but now they may also have to rely on social technology.

The great movements of the nineteenth century within medicine were the rise of bacteriology, the conquest of pain through anaesthesia and the rise of cellular pathology. But the greatest change of all, which is now beginning to affect medical and much other thinking, was the revolution induced by Charles Darwin in his *Origin of Species by Natural Selection*. The profound effects of his thought have carried on for over a century, and yet he is scarcely taken into consideration in discussions of the central themes of medicine and its place in society. A further, much lesser, change came with the institutionalisation of medical education and the accountability of doctors to the public at large as well as to their individual patients.

Pasteur was Professor of Chemistry at Lille, a wine-growing area in northern France. He found that wine and milk turned sour because of micro-organisms. He founded the science of bacteriology. It is interesting to note that he needed the problem, and the technology, as well as the genius, to solve it. The problem arose from his immediate environment which posed a practical problem, and many of the most significant scientific discoveries come from this kind of approach. But he could have done nothing without chemistry, both inorganic and organic, without the microscope and without biological stains. Again there is the sight of the genius able most fully to use the materials at hand. The genius is the ability to consider ideas outside the prevailing ethos, to speculate and go beyond what others have thought.

It is of interest that this first major breakthrough harks back to the very beginnings of thinking about disease, for bacteria are attackers from without. They might almost be said to be the supernatural powers against which primitive man armed himself with magic. At least they appear to be the inheritors of that ancient tradition. Although Pasteur's earliest work was on fermentation, he was quickly involved with the unravelling of disease in silkworms, which can suffer from bacteriological diseases. He was soon entering the realms of therapy, taking Jenner's vaccination as his paradigm. Pasteur produced vaccines for anthrax in cattle and for chicken cholera. A supreme triumph came with the treatment of rabies, also by a vaccination method.

Dalton's Atomic Theory had suggested a unitary basis for chemistry. The idea had begun in Greek times, but was on the way to some sort of verification in the first decade of the nineteenth century. This kind of thinking has appealed to many throughout the ages. The philosopher Spinoza had founded his theories on monads in the seventeenth century. A unifying basis for medicine came with Virchow, whose *Cellular Pathology* (1858) brought all disease down to the level of the cell. This gave an 'atomic' theory to the study of disease.

In some ways the new departures of bacteriology and pathology held back medical progress in other fields. But this is always the way with liberating ideas. Their full implications need slow working out by lesser men concentrating on detail. The final decades of the nineteenth century were devoted to this, as more and more bacteria were discovered and categorised and their results in causing diseases characterised. And the same was true of cellular pathology as more and more diseases came literally under the microscope. There was description and classification whilst groping for understanding.

Lister very quickly picked up the ideas about bacteriology started by Pasteur and carried on by such men as Koch. Lister revolutionised the whole approach to surgery with his antiseptic system, starting with the carbolic spray, and later moving into asepsis as well as antisepsis. Surgical and obstetric sepsis at last began to come under control, and moreover the patients could be relieved of much of their suffering by the new anaesthesia. The world of surgery started into its time of transformation.

Charles Darwin is the man who straddles the century, with his original thinking, and scientific justification of his thought. Suddenly, almost, the world had to take account of time and process in a way that it had not had to do before. It is true that there were many forerunners holding some aspects of evolution in mind. It had been thought that there was a Scale of Being right from very early times. Linnaeus had classified this scale as early as 1735. It still remains the basis of taxonomy. Lyell in his *Principles of Geology*, a book which Darwin took with him on the *Beagle*, had seen the importance of time and change in rock formations and many features of the face of the earth. Alfred Russel Wallace had developed a theory of evolution of living beings at about the same time as Darwin. The idea of evolution was in the air, and it was due to be given concrete form by someone. But it was the genius of Darwin that did so. Just as Pasteur's work was seminal and needed working out in its implications, so did that of Darwin. There was first the enraged reaction from critics that the species was not fixed, and this anger was increased when it was realised that this applied to Man just as much as to the lower animals. Man was still at the head of the ladder, but he was never again to appear as the special creation of God. It was a bitter blow to pride and the educated world reeled under it, writhing and twisting to escape the implications. But the facts were there and still are, and although there are still some who would deny the essential truths of evolution, just as there are flat-earthers denying Galileo and the subsequent galaxy of astronomers, they are now very few.

Time, change and flux came in with a vengeance. Dynamism was imported into a previously more or less static living world. It is strange now to realise that this theory caused such an upheaval. It shows how far we have moved from the attitudes of previous centuries, and especially how far we have come from the relatively simple views based on Newtonian physics. Even in that subject, Darwinism introduced a new dimension of thought, after its years of success in interpreting the world, for matter as well became mutable. It paved the way for psychology, for thinking about the mind had been previously compounded with the ideas of spirit and soul, which belonged to God. But having put Man's feet securely in the generality of living beings, even though his head might be in heaven, nothing was immune from the investigations of science. So it has proved and it continues. And once psychology was on the move so was sociology.

It is valuable to see most of the phenomena of living things in the context of individual or species set in an environment. It informs every day of work in the biological laboratory, in social work and in medicine. Nothing like this revolution in thought has come before or since. It has worked its way into every facet of life and the action and reaction that go with it.

It is probably true that Darwinism could not have come into being at any other time in history. It was the inheritor of so much that preceded it and on which it depended. It needed much that had been discovered previously in physics, chemistry, the life sciences, even in navigation, astronomy and geology. And suddenly so many of the strands were pulled together and a cloth could be woven. There is an evolution in thought, just as there is in living beings, and now it is known in the physical world too, with its changes in radio-active decay producing different elements, with its variation in isotopes and with its ever-changing particles at the heart of matter, where it becomes difficult to know whether there are particles, waves or fields of force. And the concepts go further in the postulation of an inverse world of anti-matter. It is for continuing speculation whether this would all have been possible without the enormous change in the climate of opinion wrought by Charles Darwin.

The twentieth century was therefore ushered in not only with the paraphernalia of patiently gathered facts in science and technology, but a brand new framework of thought into which to put them. It was this remarkable concatenation that led to the achievements and failures of this present century. Its failures have been largely in the human sphere rather than in its science and technology. This may be because materialism in its full implications, deriving from Newton, has not been fully modified. That would not be so surprising since its successes have in some senses been magnificent. But the reaction to materialism is building up. A new framework is needed, a new philosophy. There is a feeling of groping towards it, but it will not come. The unifying concept is wanted once more, pulling the strands together, for the weaving of a different cloth. Newton, Darwin and then who? The physical and the biological sciences have had much of their say, though there is still more to come; is it now the turn of sociology? It would certainly seem that it is in the relationships between man and man and between Man in his groups, with their conflicting ideas and cultures, that we need progress. What are the factors which lead to reconciliation? If they can be known can they be put into effect? The philosophy of materialism, still, in effect, held by so many may not be a suitable environment in which a new approach might be developed. But perhaps even materialism will work its way out of the terrestrial scheme of things. There is no reason to believe other than that all ideas, all philosophies, all schemes, live their time and die, to be replaced, it is hoped, by something which better fits human nature of the time. Even in this there is witness today that the Victorian belief in inevitable progress is not yet shaken off.

5

Mind returns to Medicine

The twentieth century saw the end of the Victorian era, the transition phase of Edwardianism, and two world wars, which engulfed almost all of the activities of the Western world. They ushered in vast social and technological changes, the effects of which still continue. They affected medicine just as much as many other areas of human endeavour.

At the turn of the century, the major impact for medicine, seen in retrospect, was that of Freud and his followers and colleagues. The sharp external static world of materialism was dissolving, partly because of Darwinism. The hold of religious conservatism had been loosened a little more. Nothing was any longer sacrosanct. Everything could be questioned and investigated. Primitive Man may have been unable to separate the mental from the material. The Greeks seem not to have distinguished greatly between the gods and Man but Christianity separated Man's divine nature from his human one, and managed to include soul and spirit as well as mind within him. Descartes put Mind and Body asunder. Darwin diminished Man's divinity severely. Freud and his school started the process of putting mind back into human affairs, and lowered the divine part of humanity still further. As in the past, the religious aspects, here the soul and spirit, were simply ignored. The emphasis on sexuality in Freud seemed to debase Man even more. Havelock Ellis began this process in 1897 when the first part of his *Psychology of Sex* was published. Freud promulgated his *Three Essays on Sexuality* in 1905, and both he and Ellis continued their writings into the 1920s. Now the cult of sex is raised almost to the status of religion. It is as if Man cannot bear the bases of his actions to be other than so elevated.

Although it has taken fifty or sixty years for Freud's impact to be fully taken into the practice of medicine, the bringing together once more of body and mind has allowed individuals to be seen whole. This, in its turn, has meant that each person is now looked at in his environment – physical, psychological and social. It is seen that Man is only Man because of these relationships. This is a final vindication of Darwinism, for Man is fully within nature, which is, in no sense, 'external' to him. Practical issues in medicine of this kind of thinking have been the growth of community medicine as a discipline, changes in family practice, and of social work of all kinds. A patient is no longer a person who can be considered in isolation from all his surroundings. Whatever these are they have a bearing upon his dis-ease. There has even been a swing away from the use of the word 'patient', and those who consult a doctor or a health services worker seem to have become 'clients'.

A further offshoot of understanding the wholeness of Man within his total context has been the increasing concern with the physical environment. This manifests itself in anxiety about pollution and over-population, and also about its visual properties and noise. In advanced countries at least it is felt that the aesthetic qualities of life must not be ignored in the fashioning of the man-made environment. Ugly buildings, unpleasant roads, noisy and inelegant vehicles should not be allowed to disfigure the landscape. It is almost as though it is recognised that Man has a soul! and that he does not live by bread alone. But this attitude seems more based in humanism and hedonism than in Christianity.

The rate of change in the twentieth century in all spheres – political, social, scientific, technological, medical – seems probably to have increased over that of the end of the nineteenth century. The new background ideas have been liberating for such progress. The methods and technology of science have been codified to a large extent, and they have been extended because of their incorporation into education. Scientists have re-produced their kind exponentially so that it is now often affirmed that there are more scientists alive today than there have ever been on the earth before. Man never seems to be able to do anything by halves. He must push what he deems to be progress to its extreme limits, and pour resources into it. It is only slowly that he comes to learn of the unfortunate results of this whole-hearted activity, which he often does painfully, that he adjusts his thinking and tries to redress the implications and actuality of what he has been doing. This is one of the messages of Sir Karl Popper. A plan is worked out, a decision is taken and a policy is put into action. Some of the plan works out more or less as envisaged, but there is always something else which was not foreseen which spins off from the policy. However careful the planning was, this is inevitable. In bad planning the spin-off may be so undesirable that it is best to abandon the original plan. More often the plan needs adjustment and modification to take account of the side-effects. It is a pity that so many planners, and those affected by them, rarely recognise these facts overtly. There are those who are so worried that they must try to foresee everything that they may therefore stultify any action at all. There are others still who lack prudence and jump to put every new idea into action without proper forethought. In any human activity of worth, some mistakes are inevitable. They cannot be eliminated at the outset. Everything in the future is in the nature of an experiment. A plan, a hypothesis, a theory selects possibilities from future likely events, and only as the future becomes the present can it be seen which of the possibilities is coming into being and which have been lost or discarded, and which were entirely forgotten from the first.

In politics, the Labour Party in Britain was founded in 1906, and it and its ideas of social relationships have increasingly been accepted by a majority of the people. The party's rise to power has been carried along by and reinforced by the trade unions. In 1913 the unions were allowed by Act of Parliament to contribute to political party funds. The ideas of trade unions proceeding from the brotherhood of man and degenerating to group protectionism have now been imported into medicine, where originally they were alien, and have become a factor in the methods of delivery of health care, for doctors now band together in formal or informal unions. Similar groups come from among the other health-care workers too.

In 1903 Mrs Pankhurst was active in the suffragette movement, and she exemplifies the growing awareness of women of themselves, of their status and place in society. It has taken them a further seventy or so years even to obtain equal pay for equal work with men, and the force of the movement is not exhausted yet. There can be no doubt that ideas on women's rights, extending back through a century or more, have changed the make-up of society and its direction, making it aware of yet another under-privileged group.

In the years before the First World War of 1914 to 1918 tertiary educational possibilities increased with the founding of Liverpool, Leeds, Sheffield, Bristol Universities and the University of Wales. The Workers' Education Association began in 1903. Newspapers for the populace were the *Daily Express*, started in 1900, and the *Daily Mirror*, started in 1903. Although fought so far away, the Boer War, which ended in 1902, seems to have given a fillip to many new ideas, and altered attitudes. There is good evidence that this nearly always happens when a country is involved in a major war. It heightens awareness of the integration of society, so that it may achieve its ends, and especially it draws attention to the human base of workers on whom society rests.

Surgery gained some ground because of the use of anaesthetics. The various body cavities could now be surgically invaded, and to some extent sepsis could be controlled by the principles of asepsis and antisepsis. But still this was an era of simple surgery which could often be practised by anyone with a medical degree, and in homes and nursing homes. Just as Queen Victoria accepting the use of chloroform in childbirth helped anaesthesia to become respectable, so did Edward VII help surgery when Sir Frederick Treves took out his inflamed appendix in 1902. And this demonstrates too that pathological investigation and diagnosis were proceeding in their classification and understanding of disease, because previously the important role of the appendix in acute abdominal inflammations had rarely been suspected.

Medicine still had to wait for its turn to burgeon. For many diseases there was little it could do in a practical, therapeutic sense, but with the aid of pathology it was able to define the natural histories and prognoses of several maladies. The seeds of endocrinology were being sown. In 1908 it was shown in Germany that endometrial changes within the uterus were physiological during the menstrual cycle and not due to abnormality and disease. Sir Henry Dale investigated pituitrin in 1909.

The effect of the war of 1914–18 on medicine was perhaps not as great as that of the later war, but it ushered in great social changes. Traumatic surgery gained some knowledge, of course, but the problems of haemorrhagic shock and sepsis were not yet conquered, although some progress was made in the use of transfusion. But the war brought an increasing understanding of medical and nursing organisation, for hospitals and field ambulance units were essential to bring immediate care to the wounded as near as possible. Socially, it was the uniting of the country towards achieving an objective that was perhaps the most notable change, including women on a larger scale than ever before. They were especially brought into the munitions factories, but also drove trucks and cars, and took on a variety of jobs previously deemed suitable only for men. An outcome of this in 1918 was the Representation of the People Act which gave the vote for the first time to $8\frac{1}{2}$ million women over the age of thirty, and for the first time too women were allowed to sit as members of Parliament. The one elected was Lady Astor.

Also in 1918 an Education Act raised the school-leaving age to fourteen years and abolished fees in elementary state schools. Before this time there had always had to be some parental contribution, however small, to children's education. The anxiety about the welfare of children extended to the introduction of school medical inspections, a hint of the growing interest in preventive medical care. Again, this was not a totally new idea. Ballantyne, in Edinburgh in 1902, had obtained the use of two beds for ante-natal care. His intention was to try to prevent congenital abnormalities rather than to care for mothers in their own right. It is interesting to reflect that no real progress was possible in this prevention until Gregg, in Australia in the 1940s, demonstrated that rubella contracted in pregnancy could cause abnormality in the fetus and newborn. It may be that Ballantyne was influenced by the publication of Mendel's work on genetics in 1900. And here it is worth noting that Mendel had originally published in 1866 but the significance of his work was not recognised; another example of the fact that a new idea needs the right climate of opinion in which to be accepted. It was not there in 1866, but it was in 1900. It is surprising now that the connection between Mendel and Darwin was not recognised in the last decades of the nineteenth century, but there would seem to be a limit on what can be assimilated in the way of ideas at any one time. Particularly, it takes time to connect one idea with another. It takes genius to recognise the connection of ideas formerly held to be disparate, and it causes a sense of shock at first in lesser minds. Overcoming this takes time, until the new idea is incorporated into culture.

During the war, in 1916, Einstein developed and published his work on the general theory of relativity. This took a new look at the relationships of space and time. He welded them together, but his revolutionary ideas have not yet worked themselves into any general climate of opinion, and though they may have altered the view of the world held by physicists there is little impact yet elsewhere. It may be that his thoughts are waiting to be incorporated into all thinking, just as Darwin's have been. Darwin's were perhaps simpler for all to understand and they took about a hundred years to capture men's minds. Einstein's may take even longer, but may be no less important.

The inter-war years are sufficiently close for them to be fairly well known. They are marked by a sense of euphoria after the release from war. They were characterised by moves to hedonism. Broadcasting by wireless and television, the motor car, mass entertainment by films and dancing all became popular. The sombre background was one of labour unrest issuing in the General Strike of 1926 and the financial crash on Wall Street of 1929. There was the gathering storm of war with the abhorrent political systems of fascism and nazism; whilst the precepts of Marx and Engels came to some practical fruition in the revolution in Russia with repercussions elsewhere. The

Spanish Civil War began in 1936, and one offshoot of this was a better understanding of the principles of traumatic surgery, especially in immobilisation of injured parts and the restoration of the blood volume by transfusion. Sulphanilamide was discovered in the same year. A new therapeutic era began.

The war of 1939–45 had its horrors, but there can be little doubt of its beneficial impact on medicine. When all are bent on one objective and there is a generated *esprit de corps*, many achievements are possible. Resources can be directed to where it is thought that they are necessary. Sacrifices of one thing to another are made without cavil and dissent. Nobody doubted that Hitlerism and the Axis powers must be defeated, and that this end must be pursued ruthlessly. The ruthlessness was finally demonstrated by the dropping of atomic bombs on Hiroshima and Nagasaki, names which have burned themselves into the conscience of the world. But it was right at the time, or seemed so to those most involved. It demonstrates the hold that cultural ideas have on the masses of the people. Warring ideologies can be carried to alarming excesses, giving another example that Man never foresees the final results of his actions. It is only when they become actual that he can comprehend them, and even then his comprehension is only partial.

It is one of the contrasts of Western society that, when most of its effort is hell-bent on destruction of its opponent forces, there is another movement of caring and concern for its members. It is perhaps not entirely surprising for it is part of group psychology. Whilst the external face deals with the outside threat, the internal face sees the relationships of the society more clearly and generates a feeling for its more underprivileged and those who will carry on its future when the holocaust is over. So not only was society directed to destruction, it turned its attention to the wounded, the mothers and children, the poor, the aged, and diseased. Social and technological resources were put into these areas as much as into the more overt purposes of war.

The military medical services have always been recognised within the armed forces as being essential to the morale of the fighting men. Few can contemplate death with equanimity, though usually sudden death is less abhorrent than maiming or lingering death. Medical services on or near the battlefield give the reassurance of swift relief. Morale may be more important in support of the armed forces than actual achievement in the saving of lives by the medical services. Since military and naval surgery have a very long tradition indeed, extending over several millennia, there may be a message here of importance in the consideration of the role of medicine in the civilian population in peace-time.

Alexander Fleming had discovered penicillin in 1929. But the world did not see its significance until the war. At the turn of the century, Ehrlich had hoped for magic bullets which would kill off invading bacteria, and a little progress had been made with arsenicals. Sulphanilamide had come into clinical practice in the years after 1936, and it needed the impetus of war to force the pace in the application of penicillin to infections consequent upon wounding. In doing so a new phase in therapy opened up. The message was learned very quickly, for suddenly, because of the almost miraculous effects of penicillin, every disease seemed potentially curable by some chemical means or other. The pharmaceutical firms turned to with a will and now new drugs poured on to the market. Pharmacology, long a rather Cinderella subject in universities, took wings. Cellular metabolism had to be intensively studied in an attempt to find chemical substances which could modify changes going on in aberrant diseased cells, or which could stimulate and support defence mechanisms. Immunology became of immense importance. Much had been known of it in infective diseases and in blood transfusion, but now its significance in many disease processes was recognised. It raised fascinating questions of how the body decided what was 'self' and 'not-self'. These arose from trying to understand how invasions from without were dealt with, but soon, in the course of many investigations, it was realised that there were problems arising from within the body which had an immunological basis. Parts of the body could be at war with other parts, and not only was this seen in the obvious case of cancer, but also in the previously ill-understood maladies now gathered together as auto-immune diseases. And one result of this thinking and discovery is that new avenues have been opened up in thinking about pregnancy and transplantations of various sorts. Such is the effect of these thoughts that universities and other bodies set up teams and departments of clinical pharmacology and clinical immunology, whilst the role of pharmacological laboratories and pharmaceutical firms has vastly increased.

The search for new effective drugs is now intense and because of technological progress foresight can be used to determine which sorts of chemical configurations are most likely to be of value. In the past thousands of drugs had to be tried on an empirical basis in the hope that one might be found which was efficacious. Ehrlich investigated 606 substances before he found salvarsan to treat syphilis. Now, because of insight into cellular metabolism and into chemistry, there is an increasing chance that once a biological chemical process can be defined, a compound can be devised and manufactured which can interfere with and modify that process. It is an astonishing revolution in thinking and technology.

Because of air attacks the battleground of the 1939–45 war was not in some far distant field. The arena of war was the whole of Europe and much of Asia. For the first time civilians were directly involved in the possibilities of sudden death and mayhem. The medical services, particularly civilian hospitals, were not geared to this kind of activity. In the main their resources were based in charity. There were government subsidies for some of them, organised by the Ministry of Health in Britain, and several local authorities ran their own hospitals. But the enemy bomber was such a threat, particularly to the larger conurbations, and charitable funding so dried up that government simply had to take over the organisation of medical care to ensure its continuance and equitable distribution. However good the military, naval and air forces were, their efforts would have been rendered vain if the civilian population had capitulated to air attack and gassing. The population was therefore dispersed as far as possible by evacuation, and just as with the armed forces they had to be given the moral support of adequate medical services. The take-over of these was complete, because it had to be. The hospitals never recovered their charitable private status after the war. There was never a chance that they could after such an upheaval. Moreover, the charitable impulse was in decline and was almost moribund for a time. The organisation of health care had changed for good in Britain, and the change has had repercussive effects around the developed world.

It has already been pointed out that a society involved in such a total war effort shows a need to look to the future as well as to the present. Children were made as safe as possible by evacuating them to country areas. Special attention was paid to expectant mothers, and the war gave a fillip to ante-natal care, and increased the tendency to hospital delivery, whereas previously the majority of births had taken place at home or in nursing homes. Rationing had become essential because of the diminution of imported food caused by the war at sea. This concentrated attention on nutrition, with special arrangements being made for children, expectant and nursing mothers, and those in heavy industry. This came close to forging a communist society, giving each according to his need. And it was largely accepted, not because of legislation and governmental force, but because the necessity for it was seen and understood by the vast majority of the people. A society forced to have unity of purpose, because of outside threat, is generally cohesive. But later experience shows that that threat has to be easily identifiable, even personified. The less differentiated threats of economic breakdown and cultural collapse do not have the same compulsion. Moreover, the weapons needed to win a war are also immediately obvious, but those needed to overcome threats emanating from social systems are debatable. Debate in a democracy can be an excuse for drifting inaction, and often is.

As with previous wars the problems of the under-privileged in society were underlined. The happy spirit pervading the country, when all were bent to one easily identifiable goal, highlighted the defects of the social system. The Beveridge Report analysed some of these and suggested a new order taking care of welfare, unemployment, health and education, as well as birth and death.

Health was seen to be the right of all who lived in a caring and well developed society. The war had irrevocably altered the pattern of the delivery of hospital care and placed it firmly in government hands. The money expended on the hospitals was so great that only government in the foreseeable future could possibly afford to support them. The result was the inauguration of the National Health Service which came into being in 1948 after the Act had been passed in 1946. There was some safeguarding of private practice, where the patient pays the doctor directly for his services, because hospital consultants could elect to work only part-time in the hospitals, and because family practitioners did not accept salaries for their services. Instead they contracted to look after a number of patients for each of whom they received an annual fee. But despite these modifications to the original intention of the legislators, wrung from them by the doctors, the basis of the delivery of medical care had changed irrevocably.

6

Paradoxes in Medical Thought

Until the National Health Service in Britain began there had been no previous systematic attempt to bring comprehensive medical care to a whole population in the Western world. Before that time each individual had to seek his own care when he felt the need for it. Although there was a large contribution from charity for many of the poorer people, usually some payment had to be made by the patient, even if only a token one. Perhaps most, however, had to pay the full costs of their medical attention or go without it, unless they were prepared to have a lesser form of service in self-medication or be charitably cared for. This system, still extant in many parts of the world, rations the use of medical resources. They are available to those who can pay for them, and less available to the others. This is medicine in the market-place, which has some merits. The patient has some responsibility for deciding when he needs medical care, and within limits he can decide where he will go to get it. The best medical care will tend to be in the large conurbations, for it is there that the money is, both because that is where the richer people make their livings and where charity funds can be collected in sufficiently large amount. Naturally, the doctors congregate there, where their services are most in demand, and as a group they are then able to press for increases in technical resources such as buildings, equipment and back-up services for diagnosis and treatment such as radiology, pathology, physiotherapy, nursing and so on.

The market-place pattern of medical care is altered when social values bring their influence to bear. These values, in the developed world, imply the right of everyone to obtain the best medical care available. Moreover, in the Western world, it is expected that these will be of the highest class and recognised as such internationally.

The foregoing chapters have been an attempt to define some of the patterns of medicine and society in the very broadest outline. Now is the time to try to draw these threads of thought together to see what the present pattern is. In previous discussion it has been suggested that no ideas are totally lost. They may be submerged in the prevailing climate of opinion, and may surge upwards once more when it changes again. The climate of opinion obviously varies from place to place and from period to period, so that the strands of thinking about medicine will vary in different cultures and find different practical expressions in the methods of delivery of medical care. The strands of thought will be given different values according to the previous history of a given society and the pressure groups within it, and according to the resources which that society will make available to its people for health. The resources allowed will be dependent upon the value accorded to medical care and so they are culturally determined too. Medicine is a part of society and is subject to conflicting ideas of its value in relation to other socially desirable aims.

British medicine has progressed probably farthest along scientific, technical and social roads and so is a suitable paradigm for analysis, for it may have lessons for those not so advanced on the journey. It is possible to see what are the underlying factors motivating medicine today in Britain, and what are the assumptions on which it appears to be based. If this is done it might be seen which of the assumptions are valid and which are not. This may give both a diagnosis and a prognosis for medicine. Prognosis is valuable for it limits expectations. Unrealistic expectations conduce to frustration and neurosis, which are probably best avoided both in individuals and societies, and groups within societies. They lead to tensions which can be minimised and made bearable. It was the utilitarians who believed in the principle of the greatest good of the greatest number, and that the motivation of the individuals and of society was and should be to increase pleasure and diminish pain. Perhaps it is within this kind of social philosophy that modern medicine must find its place.

It is worth a digression into some underlying concepts of biology, before moving once more on to the social scene. The old science of anatomy proceeds by the cutting up of the dead in order to try to reconstruct theoretical ideas on how the living body functions. It identifies systems, organs and tissues and finally cells. These can be further 'dissected' nowadays by electron microscopy, and increasingly by chemical and physical methods to find out what processes are going on. Finally it might seem that life could be 'reduced' to physical and chemical phenomena, and ideally it might be found to be simply a matter of electron and other atomic particle behaviours. But this is, in fact, not what happens at all. At some point in the dissection life goes out of the system. An appreciation of atomic particle behaviour does not predicate the existence of life unless life is already known. It appears that it is the particular organisation of the physical and chemical components which distinguishes life. It is organisation which is lost in ever more minute dissections. And the Scale of Being leading up to Man seems to be characterised by ever-increasing complexity of organisation. This is what is meant by evolution. Along the road of evolution mind makes its appearance, and this paves the way for society.

If society is dissected down to the individuals of which it is composed, and they are isolated from their interacting relationships, society disappears. As dissection proceeds down to systems, organs, tissues and cells the individual disappears, and carrying on to physical and chemical dissection causes the disappearance even of cells. But the deepening analysis is intended only for later synthesis, which leads to understanding. It is well known that both analysis and synthesis partially answer what happens and how it happens, but not why it happens. Why things happen the way that they do is so far beyond our limited comprehension, and this remains true even when some force is introduced from outside the known scheme of things, whether it is God or some life principle. These seem to have been firmly rejected as bases for many actions in the developed world at least.

The principle that seems to underlie these complex biological organisations is self-protection. This is achieved by adaptation of the system to changes occurring both within and without, and it is a matter of observation that relatively small changes allow for adaptation, whilst large changes may be overwhelming and they may cause disintegration, which is death. The struggle for self-preservation is inexplicable. It is inherent in biological mechanisms.

In addition to self-protection the organisms as individuals preserve their organisation intact by reproduction. Organisation of process cannot be indefinitely preserved in the individual, but there is some hope of doing so in the species. The exemplification of organisation in the individual breaks down when it dies, but the process within the species continues and is preserved in offspring.

These general principles of biology seem to be carried over into psychology and sociology, but this may only be because they can only be understood in this way. Understanding may be limited by our climate of opinion. But, accepting this, it may perhaps be said that a person only has a psychology because he is within society. Except for brief periods individuals cannot remain in isolation, even though there are some rare instances of this happening. The norm is for groups of people, organised into a society, to be self-protective and reproductive.

One of the reactions of society in its efforts to minimise change and strains in its relationships is division of labour. This is how medicine-men and nurses as well as other professions and occupations have arisen. And when societies are sufficiently large the various groupings become institutionalised and form societies within society, which tend to preserve the same patterns of self-preservation and reproduction. There seems to be no end to this constant proliferation. And just as there are tensions arising between individuals within a society, which require resolution so that the organisation may be preserved, so the societies within a total society develop tensions between them.

Each group develops aspirations, based frequently on unspoken assumptions, which conflict with the aspirations of others.

It is time then to ask what are the aspirations of medicine seen as a society, and what are those of society in general. This is over-simplification, of course, since there is no society in general. It is made of several smaller societies, and even within medicine there are smaller societies too. Moreover, individuals within a group cannot for all purposes be identified with that group. All belong to many different groupings, and the generally held opinions within them may logically conflict. But such is the influence of a group upon its individuals that loyalty to the ideas of one group may outweigh at any one time the inconsistencies held in a single person's mind. In this we demonstrate the influence of our psychological environment on the ways in which we think at any given moment, and this allows us to sink and keep out of sight those ideas which we might hold elsewhere at a different time. But for an analysis the shifting kaleidoscope must be held still for a moment. Differences must be submerged so that generalisations can be made. It may be unsatisfactory, but there is no other way for a finite mind to proceed.

Medicine has gathered impetus over the last hundred years. It has been impelled probably by a desire to help the rest of society and partly by curiosity, a desire to know, to comprehend, and put its discoveries into practice. The two impulses are mixed in different proportions at different times in different individuals and groups. But it is probable that it is curiosity which has the upper hand at the present time. This is shown by the increasing emphasis on research. It is culturally accepted that further research will solve all our problems. On this basis appeals are often made to the public asking them for support. The most successful appeals are those for cancer and for children. This is because they have emotive force. The emotion springs presumably from something deep in group psychology, and the underlying assumption seems to be that nobody should be allowed to die from a cancer or suffer because of this disease, and children should not suffer and die. This emotional reaction is understandable, seen from our present-day viewpoint, but perhaps it should be asked why we feel this way.

Is it the intention of medicine and of society to keep all cancer patients and all children alive? It certainly seems as if that is the unspoken assumption. It is scarcely realistic. The one certain fact about life is death, which cannot be staved off indefinitely. If it could be, then soon it would be necessary to stop all reproduction, whilst the population went on ageing. Death is a fact, and it is probable that in rational thinking we would never wish to eject it from the scheme of things. It is death which allows of freshness and renewal, not of individuals, but of Man as a species. Each new generation brings its variations and mutations and makes new adaptations to the environment possible. These may be dubbed progress, but they could be regress. Hope is on the side of progress, even though the goal of progress may not be discernible.

On the surface the aim of medicine appears to be the banishment of death, though of course that is not its only aim. Everyone knows that the aim is unrealistic and cannot be achieved, nor would it be desirable to achieve it. What, in fact, is medicine therefore doing? It is in answering this question that its basic motivations may emerge. Perhaps they are best expressed by the old motto 'To cure rarely, to relieve sometimes, to comfort always'. It has been a guide for centuries, but the therapeutic explosion has apparently changed the first to read 'To cure often . . .' Increasing successes have led to the seductive thought of 'To cure always . . .' It is in this that medicine and society have so far failed to consider the consequences of putting such an idea into action.

Research is often justified, especially to the lay public, on the grounds that its outcome will be a saving of lives. Only rarely is the question asked as to why we should want to do this. To ask it is almost heresy. There is some evidence that what is needed for the good of Man as a whole is fewer lives on this planet, so that its resources may be conserved. But medicine is a denial of this way of thinking. It seeks to maximise longevity and to help each life to be lived more fully. Curiously, just as medicine is largely accepting some of the ideas of Darwinism, in seeing the individual whole within his environment, it is at the same time rejecting a view of Man as a species in which the individuals as such matter very little. They are born, they reproduce and they die, and there are always plenty more to fill their places. No one person can exactly fill the place of another. Genetic variation and the uniqueness of each environment see to that. But the essence of life so far has been that it is just this infinite variation which has been valuable and successful. The practice of medicine denies it. It is a major paradox.

Attempts have been made to escape the dilemma by shifting ground with regard to evolution. Biological evolution proceeded according to a plan, whose main outlines have been drawn. The advent of Man brought the new dimension of psychosocial evolution in which he could now apparently direct where he was going. It is a fine theoretical idea, which ignores the practical difficulties of obtaining a consensus opinion about the goals towards which Man should head. Cultural values and local resources vary so much geographically and through time that the millennium is not yet in sight, though that is not to say that it is impossible. But all the evidence so far is that Man is far more concerned with short-term goals than long-term ones. Every treaty, every conference, every trade agreement shows that as one or other of the partners to agreement find the agreement not working to their advantage in the short term, they break it, however good the long-term consequences for all may appear to be. When it comes to trying to reach agreement on much more fundamental issues of the philosophy of what should guide Man over the next centuries, consensus is unrealistic.

It has recently been realised that a country with poor resources is probably best not to try to import high-technology medicine. It costs too much and achieves too little. It is often better to deliver care to a large part of the population than to concentrate it on a few. So have arisen the concepts of producing health-care professionals of a lower grade than those deemed to be necessary in an advanced country. They are best known as 'feldshers' in Russia or 'barefoot doctors' in China. They take what is known about medicine and apply it. They are not concerned with research, and so advancing the subject.

Medicine in the developed countries, however, increasingly concentrates on research. The reason for this is often given as the saving of lives. As previously argued, this has little basis in reason. It is more likely to be something else. Since many professionals recognise that much research is trivial and directed to no specific purpose, the reasons for research do not necessarily lie in the public good. The excuse then is that no one can foresee the ultimate good of any particular piece of research, and this is true. But is that a justification for all research? So, much research is done for the benefit of those who pursue it. Some of them are curious and just wish to know about certain aspects of the world about them. It interests them. Others do it because of the herd instinct, and they go along with the philosophy of the age, even though it may be outworn. Some do it as a stepping stone to a better career. In the process these many unimportant researches have generated a large secondary industry of published journals, exchanging facts and opinions. Despite these criticisms, however, it is probable that understanding of medical phenomena does increase overall and is made available to a wide professional audience. But there should be, and is, an anxiety that the whole process is one of taking in each other's washing and the production of valuable practical ideas is slow or non-existent. This may be because of a false idea of what science is and does. All too often it seems to be thought that the patient gathering of facts is all that is required, and then some hypothesis will miraculously emerge. But this does not happen. Popper has shown that the essence of science is not that it is verifiable, by increasing induction, but that it is falsifiable. The incorporation of this thought into scientific thinking might do much to prevent the increasing proliferation of research without orientation, and without forethought or reasonable prescience as to its outcome.

The society of medicine, like all other societies, has the instinct of self-preservation. It assumes that what it is doing is valuable to society as a whole. In general, society agrees with medicine. There is therefore a tendency to increase research, practice and teaching. Teaching will be left to later consideration, since this is part of the reproductive behaviour of the society of medicine. Research, we have seen, is often for the benefit of the researcher rather than the public good, especially when pursued at a basic level. However, even this sort of research may sometimes be justified, for there is no doubt that deep thinking about and work on a specific problem may modify the behaviour of the one who does it. Such modification may well be of value to society as a whole, and to individual patients. But research generates questions and so more research, so at least one aspect of it is that of self-preservation. The problem is to recognise potentially valueless research before it begins, and prevent it starting. Unfortunately there has been such emphasis on research that everyone is expected to have a part in it. It is this attitude which has proliferated establishments and university departments, without regard to the probable outcome. This could be valuable, but is more likely not to be, when the researcher works to further his career and not dispassionately in the seeking after knowledge. Again the problem is side-stepped by suggesting that research may not be valuable in its own right, but is useful as a teaching vehicle for the student researcher. It is then a very expensive method of education. This begs the question of the value of research and of education. The answer depends very greatly on the context in which they are pursued, and the affluence of the society which forms their matrix.

The practice of medicine, apparently done for the benefit of the populace, also has elements of self-preservation within it. There are always calls for more staff, more equipment and better buildings. They are intended to bring better care to patients. Indirectly they increase the medical establishment and its supporting staff. Developments so far have always meant expansion of facilities. These have become so costly that increasingly they have to be supported by government through taxation. Other resources are proving insufficient. This source of finance inevitably brings society in general into close contact with medicine. Public opinion begins to have its impact in a way that has not been known before. It is this which calls into question the aims of medicine and whether these accord with the general aims of society.

Essentially, therefore, medicine pursues a course which is certain to bring it into conflict with other aspirations of society. Its proponents expect it to be accorded special treatment, whilst its history shows that it has no extraordinary claims on society, other than those which society is prepared to afford.

7

Relief and Comfort.
Utilitarianism

The 'saving of lives' is a small part of the job which medicine does. It is in fact hard to define what is meant by saving lives. Presumably it means that a life is saved which would soon become extinct were it not for medical intervention. It is most difficult to be sure when this happens, for the natural propensity for healing can be so great that the humble physician will not claim too readily that it was his prowess that made the difference between life and death. In certain parts of medical practice there are definite instances where medicine preserves life. They are most easily demonstrable in injury, in acute surgical and medical emergencies and in obstetrics. But by comparison with the remainder of medicine in hospital, general and public health practice these episodes are few. The fact that they catch the attention of profession and public, by their drama, should not obscure this important fact. It is partly the dramatic improvement in the care of the acutely ill, and the manifest saving of life in that area, which has tended towards the view that 'to cure rarely' can be converted to 'to cure often'. It is a matter of degree in what is accepted as being a cure, which is easy to see after an acute illness, but very difficult in chronic illness. What was acceptable as a cure in long-standing disease a decade or so ago is often no longer looked upon as such now. Expectations rise with the passage of time, so that the relief offered to a sufferer from (say) arthritis early this century might be scorned by a similar sufferer today. This has kept medicine moving on, because its past achievements are taken for granted whilst new remedies are sought and expected. And as solutions to one set of problems are found others come to the fore. They are inexhaustible. If, with Canute, some local success can be achieved in holding the waves back, they will still flow in round the sides. In the dynamic situation of life this is inevitable. The problems of disease and ill-health will never disappear, however hard we try to banish them. This fact needs more overt recognition than it has received, both within and outside medicine. Full health for everybody is unattainable, though that is only partly true depending upon the definition of health which is adopted – a matter to be returned to later.

Obstetrics is concerned with the care of pregnant and nursing mothers and their offspring. It has passed through a period of, by modern standards, appalling maternal mortality. This is now over because of its improved methods, so attention has turned to the babies. Here too there has been a gross mortality but it is being controlled. Now attention is paid to the psychology of child-bearing women and to the prevention of physical and mental damage in the fetus and newborn. It was earlier suggested that what is deemed to be significant varies at different times in different places, and so determines the sort of thinking about caring and research which is considered worthwhile. The example of obstetrics is a perfect one. There are still parts of the world where the deaths of mothers must remain of paramount concern, those of psychology and of deaths and impairment of babies being much less so. These are of importance to individual mothers and their families, but in the wider context of society deaths overshadow them in importance. In the jargon of management 'priorities must be determined' by each society. But of course the better care of mothers in preventing many of them from dying has an effect in producing more children. The mothers live longer to increase the birth rate, and if the mother is maintained in some apparent health in pregnancy her child is more likely to survive. This is important for the future of the society to which she belongs. The size of the 'local' population in some measure determines economic, commercial and military power, and the standard of living. The instinct of the self-preservation of a society is very much at work here, and obstetrics is its handmaiden. In preserving obstetrics society is also preserving itself and its adherents.

Neonatology, the care of newborn babies, is dedicated to much the same ends as obstetrics. It preserves and maintains the lives delivered to it by childbirth. It saves lives, and tries to see that those lives are not impaired by defects. The reasons for this are humanitarian, based in religion, especially Christianity, but they also receive impetus from society in its care for its future. Society's unspoken desire is to retain a place in the sun in a potentially hostile world. The ability to live beyond mere survival depends upon a society's population in large measure, and it is important that as few members of it as possible are passengers, needing continuing care and protection.

Paediatrics, in its care of older children, carries on the work, with the blessing of society. It too has humanitarian and economic reasons at its base. There is the tug at the heart-strings as well as the hard-headedness.

The treatment of the injured, more likely to be young than old, also has the same mainsprings of preservation of society's strength. Traumatic surgery saves lives and returns them to the economic workforce. The same is true of all those younger people afflicted by an acute catastrophe who can be cured, whether that is by the help of medicine or the great powers of recovery in the young.

The older age groups nowadays form by far the largest part of those needing the care of hospitals. Much of what is done for them must be classed as relief and comfort, rather than cure. As life progresses adaptation to a changing environment, internal and external, becomes more difficult, and there is slow disintegration of organisation within. That relief and comfort are the major goals can be seen in the work of a great deal of plastic surgery, oto-rhino-laryngology, ophthalmology, much of orthopaedics and neurosurgery, thoracic and abdominal surgery and vascular surgery, including that of venous varicosities. The slow move to death cannot be staved off, but the life on the way there can be made more comfortable. Much of urology and gynaecology are similarly directed more to relief from discomfort than prolonging life.

Recent major successes in medicine have been in the infectious diseases, but before that it tended to have a caring role in making life more bearable for cardiac, chest, neurological, gastro-enterological and renal patients, whilst they perhaps succumbed more slowly to the ravages of their maladies because of medical intervention. Physicians have also done much to improve the lot of those with chronic diseases such as arthritis, diabetes and atherosclerosis. And a caring role has been that of those who look after the geriatric and chronic sick patients, and the mentally subnormal.

Psychiatry is the specialty above all which is especially concerned with relief and comfort. Mental illness is often distressing both to the sufferer and to those immediately involved with the patient. It is no surprise that this is perhaps the most rapidly advancing specialty of all in present-day society, gaining an increasing share of resources of all kinds.

It is family practice, general practice or primary care, which deals directly with 90 per cent and more of the illness and disease which occurs in the community. Increasing technology has brought it some powerful tools which bring cure to some who might formerly have been referred to hospitals with their apparently life-saving propensities. But analyses of the work of general practice show that it is trying mainly to bring relief and comfort rather than being life-saving. Nowadays especially it has been shown that about one-third to one-half of those consulting a family practitioner will do so primarily on psychological grounds. And a large number of others will see him because of upper respiratory infections, dermatological disorders and gynaecological maladies. The call upon the time of the general practitioner is essentially for relief and comfort.

Medicine in the main, therefore, has its dramatic moments of life-saving, but it is essentially about comfort. A vast army of people and extremely expensive resources are poured into this function. The philosophy underlying it is perhaps expressed by the 'greatest good of the greatest number', i.e. utilitarianism which suggests that an action is good which promotes the most pleasure and minimises pain. Such action is right in the moral sense, if it promotes happiness, not only of the individual but of all those directly or indirectly affected by it. Medicine seems to fulfil some of the ideals of this philosophy and seems on this basis to have intrinsic worth. It is grounded in hedonism in the sense that it aims to diminish pain and suffering, perhaps therefore supplying a base from which more positive pleasure might stem.

Utilitarianism tries to answer the question 'what ought a person to do?' in any given circumstances. Its reply is to do that which gives the best possible consequences, not only for the person doing, but also for others affected by the action. It is not therefore an injunction for self-centred action. John Stuart Mill, one of the earliest utilitarians, saw everything in terms of the pleasure-pain principle. Happiness was the end of Man. Anything tending to happiness was therefore good. There is little need to pursue the philosophy of utilitarianism in detail. It has had an effect in politics, economics and the law and most other areas of social activity. It is not surprising therefore to find its influence in medicine, so deeply embedded in society. But although medicine seems to be a fine flower of civilisation, and of utilitarianism, the great success of medicine has now prompted questionings and doubts. Does medicine have intrinsic value? Are all its consequences desirable? Should lives be saved whatever the cost? How much is comfort and relief worth in terms of cold hard cash and resources? How important is medicine? What should it do?

The limitations on the escalation of medicine are becoming apparent. The fact that expansion is being limited has hardly yet seeped into medical and society's thinking. There is doubt in many quarters about the inevitability of the good consequences of all medicine. Conflicts between its aims and those of society are increasing. It seems time to make an appraisal. If medicine continues on its present bases, whilst society is changing its modes of thought, then collision must ensue. The result could be that medicine might change the views of society, but it is more likely that there will be an interaction between the two in which each will modify the other's thinking. Society has always shaped medicine in the past, and is likely to do so in the future. It is society which sets the goals, even when they are not explicit. Medicine is simply one of society's responses to its environment. The professionals within medicine cannot be isolated from society in general. They must be responsive, and this needs analysis both of themselves and what they are responding to. Value judgements have to be made on all sides. Inevitably these cause conflicts of opinion, but whenever such judgements are held, however tenuously, by a sufficiently large number of the public, medicine must yield. It is this which makes it imperative to decide what medicine is about so that the values important to it are not lost, for many of them must be important to society too.

8

The Inconsistencies of Medicine and Society

Although medical practice contributes in some measure to longevity by saving some lives, the evidence is in favour of longevity being due more to social circumstances than to medical practice. Death and morbidity rates were falling before there was any really efficacious medical therapy. The falls were due to better housing, education, hygiene, sanitation, water supply, control of the conditions of food supply, clothing and warmth. All of them played their part by minimising the stresses of the physical and psycho-social environment. It is the onslaughts of the external environment which in the first instance appear to be the major causes of disease. They accelerate the rate of disintegration of the organised human body, so that illness and death are commoner than they are when the external stresses are removed. With the external environment more or less controlled in affluent societies, the rate of disintegration is more determined by the inbuilt inability of life processes to maintain themselves indefinitely, except in the very lowliest forms of life, or through the species rather than the individual. This is a reason why high-technology medicine has turned its attention to cellular processes, those inward mechanisms, including genetics and immunology and cell biology in all its forms. When society's defences against outside disease forces are reasonably secure, it can, through medicine, turn to the enemy within, and develop appropriate technologies. The aim is undoubtedly to try to increase understanding of these internal mechanisms, with the intention to modify them for the benefit of individual patients.

Why does medicine try to interfere with the life processes of individuals? Are people very important? To this last question both medicine and society return the unequivocal answer yes. The reason seems to be based in Christian ethics, bound up with utilitarianism and self-preservation. Of course the origins of these beliefs go much further back into the very primitive desire to help and co-operate with members of one's own in-group. But the scale has changed. Tribes, in-groups, are no longer small. At the least society is con-considered to be nationwide, and even this is often nowadays thought to be too restrictive, so that for some purposes society transcends national boundaries and for many the whole world is society. The inter-relatedness of all societies is recognised. The actions of one have repercussions among the rest. But the belief in the unitary species of *Homo sapiens* and in his value in different places and different cultures is by no means universally held, nor with the same degree of fervour by different individuals and groups and large societies. However much it may be desired, the world is not a global village, except in the minds of a few who command the resources to make it superficially so. Whatever reason may say, the emotions bind us all more closely to the immediate circle of acquaintance than to those more distant. Cultural barriers still prevail, except in isolated instances, against the call for thinking universally.

The unexpected spin-off from the thinking and actions of advanced societies, some of which are expressed through medicine, has been the growth of population, its pressure on resources and pollution of all kinds. The prophecies of Malthus seem to have come true after about 175 years, and Darwinism for Man has come into its own. The species is out-running its means of support. A response has been to try to marshal resources to improve food supply and diminish pollution. But medicine in attempts to preserve and prolong life, even though that is not its true aim, still seems to be continuing on its course as if no catastrophe were imminent. The agronomists increase the food supply whilst the doctors busily try to enlarge the numbers of mouths to feed.

Medicine has, however, made a partial series of responses to the felt needs of society. It has applied methods of contraception, of sterilisation and abortion on a wide scale. It, and society, have tended to cloak the imperative drive for self-preservation in the apparently humanitarian ideal of every baby being a wanted baby. Arguments are adduced for making every life a comfortable life, when it is the species response which is at the base of the actions. And, of course, medicine and society are dabbling with thoughts of euthanasia. The overt motives are those of humanitarianism, but there are deeper ones at a biological level. It is the species against the individual.

With the physical environment more or less tamed, the environment of Man becomes Man himself. Action must then be taken against him. War, famine and disease, the ancient cullers of human populations, must be banished by humanitarianism and be replaced by contraception, sterilisation, abortion and euthanasia. Man culls his own domestic herds and plants, and extends this process to the wild, so it seems natural to want to turn these successful methods towards himself. But he is still rather half-hearted about it. Compunction keeps breaking in and society cannot bring itself to put these policies fully into operation. These are the evils of war, famine and disease, but it is not wholly convincing to all that these are worse than deliberate culling.

Medicine displays the social schizophrenia acutely. It seems to want to banish disease and famine from the world, and in war-time it is accorded a specially privileged role in caring for the injured, and at the same time it supplies the shock troops for the prevention and destruction of human life in population control. It has no philosophy of its own which is consistent. It leans heavily on society for its thinking and actions despite any pleas to the contrary. It is even responding to society's thinking about high-cost medical care in entertaining serious doubts about the value of medicine in all places at all times.

By far the largest expenditure in medicine goes into hospitals. They have large staffs and sophisticated equipment. Yet they deal with only about 10 per cent of the illness which is present in the community at any one time. The hospital doctors delve deeply into the life processes and try to modify them at high cost, whilst they also retain the ancient custodial role of shielding their patients from the mainstream of society. The value of doing this is becoming increasingly doubtful. The call is then to transfer the medical and other resources to where the illness is and where it should be dealt with in the community. It is assumed that dealing with illness there will be cheaper and more effective than in hospitals. This may be so, but there is evidence accumulating that such health care is self-preserving and replicative, and its costs may be just as great as those of hospital and custodial care. To perform efficiently nowadays the community doctor must have helpers such as nurses, physiotherapists, social workers, psychiatric social workers, psychologists, diagnostic services and clerical help. Just as in hospitals the health teams are self-generating. And when the backlog of present disease is apparently dealt with, the definition of what illness is changes, so that more people are pulled into the illness category. The motivating forces within medicine, the desire to feel wanted and needed, find a ready echo in society. States of unwellness are then seen by the public as disease, and for every disease there must be a cure, preferably by a course of pills, for these have been seen to be powerful and less incommoding in general than a surgical operation and hospitalisation. Medicine, then, does not diminish illness, it generates it, by changing in response to its own needs for self-preservation and replication. In this, of course, medicine is not alone. All societies within society do the same thing, advertising being the most obvious activity devoted to generating wants which become needs.

What is illness and what is health? A widely quoted definition of health is that of the World Health Organisation at its founding in 1946: 'Health is a state of complete physical, mental and social well-being and not merely the absence of disease or infirmity.' In one way and another, medicine acts as if this were literally true, even though many doctors do not explicitly realise it. If it is fully accepted then virtually the whole population is ill, and medicine can be called in to give assistance. Few people do function at that high level of health. There are headaches, rheumatism, joint pains, anxieties, fears, doubts, distress, grief, dyspepsia, rashes, eye and ear defects and a host of other minor discomforts. Should they be classed as illness and lead therefore to the delivery of some health care which always costs something? And can the aged, the chronically diseased and the maimed ever be said to be healthy? According to the WHO definition they cannot be. Moreover, life is not a state, it is a constant dynamic adjustment of the individual to his environment. Organisms and environment change from day to day, almost from hour to hour. The successful organism, the person who is well, is the one who maintains a reasonable equilibrium between himself and what goes on around him and inside him. The decision about this equilibrium is a matter of judgement, either by the individual himself, some other person or the doctor. As expectations of what constitutes health rise, the decision that something abnormal is in train is made on ever flimsier grounds.

Another sign of medicine generating ill-health is in its screening processes. Here it is intended that a disease should be recognised before it becomes a dis-ease for the patient in causing symptoms. In this way a large number of people can be turned into patients requiring medical services before they know that they do. The army needed for the detection of these hidden diseases increases. This is not wholly bad for society since it is a requirement that people should be employed in something that society deems useful. As the labour needed in primary production diminishes because of better technology, there is an increasing need for secondary industries. The health industry has mopped up large numbers from the pool of labour. In many countries it has come to rival the mediaeval church, which was a large society employing many people and generating work in the building of cathedrals and churches. In a more secular society the health industry too employs many and builds temples to Hygeia, in hospitals and health centres of all kinds.

Medicine started out because of a manifest need to help people in distress and pain. It was limited in scope and was delivered on a local basis only to those members of the in-group which it served. It became highly successful in its ability to relieve and comfort. It has come almost to believe in its potential to prevent death. There has arisen in some minds the thought that disease might be banished from the human scene, and this without the implication that if it happened it would mean the banishment of death also. No thought is given by such Utopians to the possible outcome if these thoughts could be actually realised. Medicine may banish some diseases, but will always find others. In controlling epidemic diseases and preventing them, medicine helps with the galloping increase of population, which is now thought to be such a threat. And medicine is even more paradoxical in trying to cure infertility and often succeeding. Having entered into human affairs on a simple basis the successes of medicine and other activities have led to a goal undreamed of, where Man is his own worst enemy. Yet medicine continues on its steady way, researching ever more deeply into life processes, relieving individuals, helping them to reproduce and to see that their offspring survive, generating illness so that it interferes ever more in individual lives by raising standards of health, and now it finds itself not only society's instrument of succour but its death-dealing arm. The bases of medicine are insecure and inconsistent, but no more so than those of society, but there can be no support for the idea that medicine has any claims to a philosophy independent of those of the society in which it functions. It is manifestly just one of the responses of humanity to its condition and is as inconsistent as the bases from which it sprang.

9
Medical Education

When the practice of medicine is expansionist, attracting ever more patients into its net by altering the definitions and expectations of health and illness, and looking for disease before it is symptomatically manifest, then it must multiply and reproduce. More doctors are needed, and that is the function of medical education.

In the nineteenth century in Britain, the majority of doctors were essentially general practitioners. They were often apothecaries, some of whom were apprenticed to a doctor in practice and then had a spell in what was called 'walking the wards', commonly of one of the London hospitals. Some doctors had been previously enlisted in naval or military service as surgeons. The Royal College of Surgeons evolved from the Barber-Surgeons in 1800. Physicians had usually attended either Oxford or Cambridge Universities, were members of the ancient Royal College of Physicians and practised mainly in and around London. They were the educated men of medicine who had read the classics and knew some anatomy, botany and chemistry. They diagnosed and prescribed drugs, but they did not dispense them. The tradesmen of medicine were the apothecaries and surgeons, who were often the amanuenses of physicians, though they could and did practise independently.

There were many well-known schools of medicine throughout Europe and Great Britain and the better students often travelled to universities other than their own to continue their education. But there was no royal and right road to becoming a doctor and there were few rules about entry to the profession, though the universities, the colleges and the guilds laid down some regulations and conducted examinations. The Royal College of Physicians, in particular, prescribed certain ethical codes of conduct to which its members were expected to conform. They could be disciplined by the college and could have their membership revoked. But there was little formal regulation or discipline of surgeons and apothecaries.

As so often in the history of society it was felt that such relative chaos could no longer be countenanced. Medicine was becoming too important to itself and to society. Prompted by medicine, society, through Parliament, introduced the Medical Act of 1858. There had, of course, been many previous attempts to pass Bills to regulate medicine. This one was the culmination of a series. It did not come into force without resistance and opposition. A major provision was to set up the General Medical Council for Medical Education and Registration. The Council was free of political control, and advisory rather than authoritative in its powers. It was able to license certain bodies, mainly the universities, to give various degrees and diplomas, and had power to oversee the conduct of medical education. By admitting those with appropriate qualifications to the Council's Register, and by reserving certain rights only to those on the Register, it began to formalise the practice of medicine and co-ordinate and control medical education. It curbed the increasing powers of the Royal Colleges and other licensing bodies, which at that time abounded, and it gave greater independent powers to universities. The Council was another instance of the process of institutionalisation.

A very early concern of the General Medical Council, quoting Charles Newman in *The Evolution of Medical Education in the Nineteenth Century* (p. 197), was medical education. '"When the Council originally met in 1858, there was a general feeling that the first thing to be considered was the mode of improving the general education of the student" . . . The first Committee on Education set up by the Council reported in 1859 that "no person should enter the medical or surgical profession who has not received an education in general knowledge such as will be equal, at least, to that required by the national education bodies". By these they meant the universities, and in this statement they were expressing the opinion that surgeons and apothecaries ought to be as worthily educated as were the physicians, or, indeed, the members of any profession.

'The General Medical Council defined the position in more detail in 1870 when they said: "Prior to 1858, although the education, both general and professional of . . . the higher walks of the profession was such as secured the supply of a certain number of well-educated gentlemen and accomplished practitioners, yet the strictly professional education of even those was in many respects seriously defective. But as regards the main bulk of the profession . . . the education was so defective that the profession was in danger of being overrun with illiterate and incompetent men."'

Newman makes the point that the early Council was concerned with character and general education. It therefore laid down that the preliminary examination before entry to a medical course should consist of English, arithmetic, algebra, geometry, Latin and one subject from among the following – Greek, French, German, natural philosophy, including mechanics, hydrostatics and pneumatics. However, there continued to be concern with literacy and there were complaints about the standard of this and bad spelling in the candidates of 1899 and 1920. The concern with the general education of the doctor ignored the fact of the rising content of scientific medicine. The educated Christian gentleman of yesterday, who obtained his professional expertise after his preliminary general education, was the original ideal, but this was crowded out by the requirement that the newly qualified doctor should be full of more useful knowledge which could be immediately applied in practice. At qualification the doctor could until quite recently go straight into practice without supervision, and without having to undertake any further postgraduate education or training at all. Medical education in the nineteenth century therefore had to try to ensure that the emerging graduate would be a safe general practitioner. Not only had he to be educated, he had to have the rudiments of the craft and technology of medicine at graduation. After that he was left to his own devices, but need do nothing but practise.

The advent of the General Medical Council introduced and

formalised examinations at various points in the student's career. It was thought that they were an essential part of the educational process. To avoid favouritism to candidates, and as a check on standards, the Council insisted that examiners should be appointed from outside the students' own institutions. Major examinations at set points in the medical course are not now always accepted as educationally desirable but, if they are, the principle of having them monitored by external appointees is a good one. Probably all major institutions need some form of auditing from time to time.

From the many systems of medical education of the late nineteenth century a more or less basic pattern has emerged in the English-speaking countries. It is based on the principles which emerged from the recommendations of the General Medical Council. There are, of course, many experiments in medical education being conducted, but the essentials remain the same. The problems remain the same too, probably because there is no consensus about the aims of medical education. This, in its turn, stems from the fact that there is no consensus about what medicine is and what it does and where it fits into society. If it were possible to be sure exactly what a doctor does it might be possible to structure a course which could produce him.

The nearest approach to consensus about what sort of doctors were needed in Britain came around the end of the nineteenth century. Then, nearly all doctors were general practitioners and were expected at graduation to have a practical competence in medicine, surgery, midwifery and pharmacotherapeutics. The course and the examinations were constructed to try to produce this paragon who encompassed everything medical. But knowledge has now so accumulated that this is no longer possible. Yet the opinion is still often held that the object of present-day medical education is to produce a general practitioner. In the undergraduate years at least this cannot be done unless we would be content with a different type of doctor from the one we have now. More totalitarian countries than those of the Western world have decided exactly what they want, as in the 'feldshers' of Russia and the 'barefoot doctors' of mainland China. Other less developed countries, especially in Africa, have also to consider having the same sorts of health worker. The doctor of the Western world is expensive to produce, so his numbers are relatively few, and he tends to function at too high a level for simpler, poorer communities. This means that his high expertise cannot be delivered to the whole population which is deemed to need him. The result is that poorer countries must produce a lower cost health worker in greater numbers, so that at least some health care can be delivered to the whole populace. This is on the basis that some health care is better than none, and that it is right that everyone should have access to it.

The Western world has until recently taken the view that only the very best medicine will do for its peoples. This has involved Western countries in producing more and more doctors to meet expectations. This policy is being called into question, in practice if not in theory, by the apparent need for a small army of health workers with which the doctor surrounds himself so that his high skills can be more appropriately used. The remainder of his health team have duties delegated to them. Just as medicine generated hospital specialties out of its general practice, so it is now beginning to spawn further specialties in the community. And as the general practitioner found that he could no longer be competent in surgery and midwifery and the whole of medicine, he no longer finds that he can be competent in nursing, psychology, social work and health education. These areas of practice must then be handed on to specialists in those fields. As with other groups within society these groups of specialists begin to take on a separate life of their own. They develop the same characteristics of self-preservation and reproduction as medicine. The members band together to enhance their autonomy and their rights. They try to separate themselves from others in their functions and they do not accept that the doctor controls them or has any leadership functions in regard to them. This means that more and more staff and more and more specialties intrude into health care. And as with medicine itself they generate more and more ill-health by going out to find it in the community. They raise expectations which, when they are not fulfilled, are classed as illness.

These tendencies make it increasingly difficult to decide what the function of a doctor is and therefore to define a suitable education for him. Probably only medicine can decide this, though its propositions will be subject to the over-riding control of general public opinion, which is usually propagated by parliamentary institutions and government. It is they who put limitations on the aspirations of medicine, since it is they who provide the finance for education and for medicine. It is true that in many parts of the world a large income for medicine comes from outside government sources mainly by insurance or private fees but this proportion is declining and as medicine comes to cost more and more it is inevitable that only government finance can bear the greater share of the burden.

Modern medical education seems to proceed on certain assumptions. The first is that medicine is a good thing and that it will go on expanding its scope in practice, in research and in being brought to the people. The second is that doctors must be educated so that they will be able to respond to the rapid changes in medicine which seem to be inevitable. The first assumption implies that there is no upper limit to the number of doctors which the world needs. The second determines the form and content and method of medical education. The need for doctors is a matter for later consideration. Although the 'educators' of doctors at present seem to hold the upper hand, the 'trimmers' are active. These last seem to hold to the view that the doctor is a technologist and that his functions in society are restricted and can be delineated. They maintain that much of the knowledge imparted by present education is useless for the later practitioner. They therefore ask for drastic pruning of various parts of the course and believe that the length of the course can be reduced by at least one year if not more. The apprenticeship system of medical education has an old history. The 'trimmers' would tend to revert to it for they believe that the theoretical, more academic aspects of the medical curriculum should be sacrificed so that the aspiring doctor may more quickly practise under the tutelage of one who is more experienced.

There are two parts to any professional education. They are the understanding of principles, and the crafts of putting these into practice. Alternatively, they may be seen as theory and practice. It is the proportions of these thought to be valuable which separate the 'educators' from the 'trimmers'. The 'educators' emphasise theory at first, making craft and technology a matter for the postgraduate, whilst the 'trimmers' want to get on to the craft as quickly as possible, saying that comprehension is not essential for undertaking practical tasks. They believe that all the necessary comprehension and education will come out of the craft as it is practised.

The 'educators' seek to make the undergraduate a comprehender first. Their aim is to expose the student to all the branches of medicine so that he shall understand something of each of them, what they are, what they do, how they do it and what they achieve. On this basis the student will have obtained a panoramic view of medicine by the time he graduates. Out of what he has seen and learned as a student he can then select areas for deeper postgraduate studies according to his inclination. It is assumed that this wide education in many subjects will make the doctor responsive to the changing needs of health care, and of medical progress, whatever they may be and whenever they come. They may arise either from advances within the body of medicine or from the changing attitudes of society.

The foregoing discussion of the dichotomy between the 'educators' and the 'trimmers' leaves out of account the wishes of the students and their expectations of medicine. They too have a group psychology which is essentially based on their understanding of the views of the general public and of its attitudes to medicine. Because of the increasing weight being given to student opinions they are partially influential in changing medicine, whilst on the other hand the students are exposed to medical practitioners during their courses who modify student opinions towards the loosely held views of the medical establishment. Students begin medicine as members of the public, and end with much of themselves absorbed into their profession as a special group.

The only really common thing about medical students at the beginning of their careers is that they are intelligent, as judged by the results of examinations, mainly in scientific subjects, studied at school. Their reasons for wishing to become doctors are as varied as they are themselves. Some have derived their ideas about medicine from members of their families who may be doctors, but most have their ideas from other indirect sources. They embrace a loosely-knit weave of folklore, television, reading and a vague aura coming from any brushes they may have had with medicine when they or relatives have been ill. This received ragbag of ideas, allied with some literacy and scant scientific knowledge, is the material which medical education goes to work on. The teachers whom the students will meet will also be as variable as themselves. They too will have disparate notions of what medicine is about and what it is that they are trying to do with the 'material' placed in their hands. They in fact teach from an inherited tradition, based very much on the historical outline of medicine given in the first few chapters of this book. There is, of course, nothing wrong in this, since there is no other place from which to start than the one in which you are. And certainly the general tradition of medicine has nothing of which to be ashamed. It has served society well, both in its own and society's eyes. Its practitioners have been very responsive to society's changing needs, have often been self-critical and have often led society's thinking. So the traditional system of medical education, developed particularly over the last 150 years, has not seriously failed at least the developed societies which it exists to serve. There would seem to be no good evidence for a totally radical revision of medical education, though that is not to say that its emphases ought not to change. Revolutionaries in this area, as in others, are ridiculous in believing that the slate can be wiped clean, so that some better order may be written. Evolution is the only course likely to gain acceptance, for the base from which change might be introduced cannot be altered.

With each generation of students medicine changes. The teachers deliver messages different from those that they received, and the students receive them and later transmit them in a different way too. Moreover, each generation of students is differently responsive to its perceived ideas of society. This is a special statement of the way in which all society changes through time. The central core of transmitted knowledge seems to remain much as it was, but it is being constantly reinterpreted, often in slight, almost imperceptible ways, so that the original core is not quite the same as it used to be. And the rate of change of the accepted core is apparently accelerating all the time.

The medical curriculum is of interest because it gives some understanding of what the generality of medical opinion believes to be the requirements of a doctor. There are many variants of the general theme of medical education but it is possible to abstract an essence of the curriculum. Physics and chemistry are the substratum of biological activity. They are needed to give understanding of the cell and of the organism. They are essential for comprehension of much research, which forms such a large part of the medical journals. In these, as in later subjects, it is realised that it is quite impossible to foretell the potentialities and aptitudes of individual students, for each is unique, so they must all be given some groundwork on which they might later build, in ways that they wish. Investigations of career choices show how these change among students as they progress through the course and as their understanding of the nature of medicine changes. In a free society this makes nonsense of any claim to know exactly what will and what will not be useful knowledge for the qualified doctor. Of course, this would change if there came any political direction of medicine. If a student could be compelled to be, say, a general practitioner in a certain circumscribed society, it would be possible to analyse exactly what was required of him and then design a training. But this ignores the fact that the society he serves will change over the course of time, and if his education is too restricted he may be unable to adapt to the changing circumstances. Moreover, he may move to work in a quite different kind of society.

With physics and chemistry there is usually an introduction to biology. It cannot be denied that the basis of medicine is rooted in biology and life processes. The problem is not whether biology should be taught and learned, but how much of it, and which branches of it, but this is true of all the subjects introduced into the medical curriculum. A benefit of biology is that it introduced a mode of thinking and a scientific cant or jargon. This use of words and their understanding is vital to later progress. It has been suggested that the vocabulary of medicine is in quantity the equivalent of that of two foreign languages, even though the syntax is that of the known language. Nevertheless there is a need to use and re-use biological terms until their meaning becomes ingrained.

Anatomy, physiology and biochemistry begin the process of concentrating on Man. It is deemed essential that the doctor should know where the organs and tissues are and how they function normally. Only so will he know the deviations from normal, the understanding of which is the ultimate aim of medical education. Anatomy is the most ancient of the sciences directly germane to the practice of medicine, and in the eyes of many has held, and continues to hold, too large a share of the students' time. There have been moves to mitigate this complaint, but despite assertions to the contrary, there can be little denial of a place for some anatomy in the education of a doctor. Some physiology and biochemistry can scarcely be denied either. It is a question of how much and in what depth.

Often along with these basic medical sciences there is an introduction of behavioural science and community medicine. This acknowledges Darwin and Freud in understanding Man psychologically and as a social being. There are those who tend to see him as only such, and they are aided by the recent growth of the army of psychologists, both amateur and professional, and the sociologists. But medicine keeps coming back to the individual person and his body, so education brings in the concepts of microbiology and pathology – the bases of disease and disorder. The emphasis changes in moving from normal Man to abnormal Man. There follows the whole host of the different clinical disciplines, seen mainly in hospital, though increasingly disease is witnessed in its community context in family practice and in the community.

The objective is to produce a doctor who has been 'exposed' to everything that medicine has to offer, whilst realising that this cannot possibly be done because of the range of disorder to which people are heir, and the complexities of the methods ued to try to remedy their ills. Inevitably there are criticisms of content and method in medical education, and of the 'kind of doctor' who emerges.

Medical education is not innovative. It follows trends which develop in medicine and society. Its history follows closely the outline of medical ideas previously sketched. At first there was only empirical practice, so making apprenticeship essential, and this extended to therapy as well as diagnosis. Botany was needed for medical treatment, and manipulative skill for surgery. A knowledge of plants and herbs is no longer required because chemistry, biochemistry, pharmacy and the drug manufacturers have made it unnecessary. They have all developed skills beyond the doctors' competence. Manipulative skill is now reserved for a few surgeons, making it unnecessary for the undergraduate. The same is true of obstetrics. Manual dexterity is perhaps desirable in its own right, but need not be specially cultivated. Now it is not certain at what stage of medical education apprenticeship should be introduced. It is expensive in its small ratio of apprentices to master, and it is valuable for skills of craft rather than for general education.

The burgeoning of biology under the impact of Darwin naturally brought this subject greatly into medical education, and as its later progress has been increasingly in the hands of chemistry, biochemistry, physics, molecular biology and genetics, these too have become incorporated in the medical curriculum. In the earlier days of these developing subjects, the medical student was expected to master some of their skills. As these have become more erudite, such mastery has become impossible. Instead, the student is now expected to have a grasp of their principles, without full comprehension of their methods. This was what happened with botany. Long after the demonstrated need of this subject for the doctor, it was still included in medical curricula. From the practice of botany, the medical student moved to only an understanding of botanical principles, and later still the subject was dropped entirely. Whether there is a general lesson here for the more modern subjects just enumerated is difficult to discern.

Anatomy certainly shows some of the trends seen in botany. It was a queen of medical sciences, reached a zenith in minutiae, which had to be learned by all students, insisted on total body dissection by them, and now is retreating from its preeminent position. The skills of anatomy are no longer required, nor are the details. Anatomical principles only are taught and expected. The specialists in anatomy are now the surgeons, and even they find that the small details of anatomy are not essential parts of knowledge for the practice of their skills.

Physiology, microbiology and pathology, all products of the end of the nineteenth century, similarly show signs of expansion, excessive detail and emphasis on method, reaching a zenith and then retreating within medical education. They too have withdrawn to the teaching of principles to the undergraduate. Psychology, sociology, community medicine, psychiatry, pharmacology, the twentieth-century additions to medicine, demonstrate the same propensities, though differing in the rate at which they progress through the different phases.

Even the clinical subjects have had to retreat in the face of rapidly expanding knowledge. The content of each specialty is large and its methods are increasingly erudite. Principles only can be imparted. To do more is over-burdening within the time available for medical education.

All this is not a special problem for medicine. It afflicts all branches of knowledge when they are rapidly expanding. What is required of the product of education, what are the principles of the subjects taught, and what the detail, will continue to be matters of debate. They cannot be resolved except by a committee of one, given supreme powers. Even with such resolution, the medical education given could not remain suitable for all students, and for all doctors wherever and whenever they might practise. There is no one doctor suited to all times and all places. It has been a fallacy of medical education to entertain this possibility. It still sometimes bedevils the thinking of some teachers, who, when they believe it, have some unattainable ideal in mind, often moulded in their own image.

10

Criticisms of Medical Education

When the aims of society are unclear, so are those of medicine and of medical education, and when each individual is so unique and holds his own views on these aims, it is scarcely surprising that hardly anyone is fully satisfied with the present mix. Almost more surprising perhaps is that there is a general consensus about medicine and medical education. But just as it seemed worthwhile to look at the usual type of medical education to try to decide if it would give a guide to what doctors were thinking about the role of medicine, so it seems that criticisms of medical education may help to decide where medicine appears to some not to be adapting to the needs of society.

A blanket criticism is that we are not producing the right kind of doctor with the present system. This presupposes that the critic knows just what kind of doctor is needed. When the speaker is a doctor himself it usually means that he would produce a doctor who is moulded in his own image, especially if he is a general practitioner. But this is parochial and makes assumptions which are not warranted. It is not possible to produce a finished doctor suitable for practice in Australia, Indonesia, India, South America, the United States, Russia, China, the United Kingdom, in rural areas, in city slums and sleek suburbs. In fact, medical education in developed countries has done quite well in its responses by providing a relatively undifferentiated product, which can later be differentiated by postgraduate training and education. In a free society it is axiomatic that the newly qualified doctor has the freedom to decide into what branch of medicine he would like to go to practise. This is the cultural ethos. It is not immutable, as Russia and China have shown. Since the production of doctors of the present type is a slow one, there is no doubt that it can be speeded up by producing specialists in smaller fields of medicine. This has been done in various forms of community and general practice by using other less expensive health care professionals. It seems highly likely that a very large number of general practitioners function at a level far below that of the potential generated by their education; that is, they use only a very small part of what they have learned, especially in the undergraduate years. In particular, their physical diagnostic skills, acquired during the undergraduate clinical years and afterwards in hospital junior posts, are comparatively rarely called into play. Surveys of Western general practices seem to show that most of the patients have relatively trivial physical complaints, often respiratory, or gynaecological or dermatological. By far the larger part of practice is related to psychological problems of varying kinds, and often consequent upon social malfunctioning. Ninety per cent of all medicine is practised in such a way, and only ten per cent of it takes place in hospitals. It is a frequent criticism that the amount of financial support flows into these two areas in exactly the opposite percentages.

If most of family practice is of this kind, does it need a doctor who is as highly educated as our modern ones? The modern trend suggests that it does not. Much preliminary care can be given by nurses and pharmacists and others. It has always been so, but of recent years patients have come to expect that it is the doctor whom they should see. They want what they believe to be the best advice and treatment. Medicine has tried to see that they do get medical care as opposed to anything less. It is now the general practitioners themselves who are calling this necessity into question. They surround themselves increasingly with supporting staff of various kinds, and in the first instance have turned, almost inevitably, to their old colleagues, the nurses. These are often asked, in general practice nowadays, to be the preliminary screen before the patient reaches the doctor, and often indeed there is no necessity for the patient to see him at all. Even after seeing the doctor the follow-up care is often handed over to the nurse. Pharmacists, psychologists, social workers often perform similar functions. It is now said that the doctor is just one member of the health care team. This has always been the case where the doctor is in hospital practice. Patients there need nurses, domestics, administrators and many others for their care. But until recently the general practitioner undertook to provide almost total medical care, with only slight help from nurses.

Now the professionals in other disciplines, such as those of sociology and psychology, draw attention to the relative ignorance of the doctor in their subjects and begin to question his value. Certainly many of them feel that he has no special rights to claim to be the team leader. His presence in the community is only a convenience for members of it, so that they do not have to travel far to obtain their medical care. But what sort of medical care do people need and is the present type of family practitioner the one needed to give it? There is no doubt that his role is changing. He has certainly given up the idea that he alone can provide a total service. Not only are there health care teams, there are teams of general practitioners. They are needed because they must pool their skills and because social changes have seemed to make it necessary for doctors to have time off from their work.

The expertise which the general practitioner alone of members of the health team can bring to the patient is that of diagnosis, especially in the physical sphere. There is no doubt that he also, in the course of practice, acquires skill in the psycho-social field, but there are others who can do just as well here, for they may believe that they are the real professionals whilst the doctor is a dabbler. The response of the medical profession to these criticisms is to try to compete with these newer professions on their own ground. Hence come the calls for an increased content of psychology, psychiatry and sociology in medical education. Perhaps this is right, but it is not self-evident. Maybe medicine is trying to do too much, and if so this brings the wheel full circle for it begs the question of what medicine is and what its content should be. It can be looked on as the whole Biology of Man, which carries the implication that anything affecting Man is the legitimate concern of medicine, or at the other extreme medicine can largely be viewed as dealing with Physical Man – Man without too much intrusion of mind and social function.

A simple scheme of things is one which looks at Man at varying levels. At the 'biological' level he is a body with cells, organs and tissues. He may be normal or abnormal in these. These can be investigated at deeper levels by the methods of chemistry and physics. Moving to higher levels of integration above the 'biological' takes one first into the spheres of psychology and then to sociology. Few would doubt that medicine is about 'biology', physics and chemistry. That is how medicine historically has grown. Most would also now accept that psychology and psychiatry are part of medicine, though as previously seen they are of relatively recent appearance. They have had some difficulty in making themselves respectable within the canon of medicine. Now sociology is having the same difficulties, and there are some within the medical profession who see this subject as no real part of the body of medicine; not too uncommonly psychology, psychiatry and sociology are referred to as 'soft options'. By its reactions, however, medicine seems to be drifting into a view of itself which makes it the Biology of Man without restriction. This would seem to be inevitable for, in considering the levels of organisation of Man, it is not possible to delineate where one level ends and the other begins. Above all it is not possible to extricate exactly the psychological from the physical and the psychological from the social. Culture and biology are one. The professionals in physics, chemistry, biology, psychology and sociology are all indeed more knowledgeable in their respective subjects than the doctors, but there is still room for the generalists which they profess to be. Jacques Barzun in his *The House of Intellect* puts the professionals in their proper place.

'That same abundance of information has turned into a barrier between one man and the next. They are mutually incommunicado, because each believes that his subject and his language cannot and should not be understood by the other. This is the vice which we weakly deplore as specialisation. It is thought of, once again, as external and compelling, though it comes in fact from within, a tacit denial of Intellect. It is a denial because it rests on the *superstition that understanding is identical with professional skill*. The universal formula is: "You cannot understand or appreciate my art (science) (trade) unless you yourself practise it"' (my italics).

This puts it in a nutshell. Medical education is about understanding a large variety of professions, not about practising them. One does not have to be able to play every instrument in the orchestra with marvellous technique to be able to conduct, but an understanding of the relationships of one instrument to the other and where they fit into the musical piece is essential. So at least in undergraduate education it is vital to resist the pressures of every professional group to impose its wishes on the curriculum. All must be kept in their place, whilst recognising that there will never be complete agreement about the proportion of each which should be included, nor in which order they should be presented, But as new aspects of the Biology of Man come to be known, some part of them should come into the medical course so that understanding may be given the chance to flourish, and this means that some parts of the course must be curtailed. It has been wisely said that knowledge not only accumulates, it becomes obsolete. The useless bits must be excised, but this demands a unity of purpose from the medical educators and a willingness to submerge their professionalisms for the good of the whole, which is unlikely ever to be quickly achieved. But there are signs that this does slowly happen. Curricula do change. It is only the impatient who suffer, and they do so because their time-scale is too short. This is an argument for introducing history into the medical course to gain long-term perspective.

THE UNIVERSITY

Prior to the Medical Act of 1858 most medical education, that for the surgeons and apothecaries, was by apprenticeship.

Universities scarcely figured at all except for the few physicians who went to Oxford or Cambridge, or universities in continental Europe. The Act tried to make medical education an education rather than a craft or trade. It has succeeded insofar as all medical education in the Western world is now university based. There are still large elements of apprenticeship in the clinical years, but the basic medical sciences are now university disciplines. Because university teachers tend to have lower incomes than practising doctors the basic medical disciplines have become depleted of the medically qualified and the departments are increasingly staffed by scientists. Those who see medicine as a technology, an applied science, deplore this and some call for making it once more a hospital-based apprenticeship. They emphasise the craft of medicine rather than its educational content. Some, on the other hand, would see the presence of scientists in the pre-clinical subjects as broadening education.

There can be little doubt that the basic medical sciences could be taught within the hospitals. There is much expertise there. But it would be of a different kind from that now taught in the universities. It would be essentially practical and oriented to practice as it is now, rather than as it may become. Hospital scientists have a different function from those in the universities. Both probably have a part to play in medical education. Over-emphasising the differences, one group looks to the future and the other to present practice.

THE HOSPITAL

It is said that medical education today is too much concentrated in the hospital. This criticism is based on the fact that most medicine is now conducted in the community, and the criticism comes mainly from general practitioners and epidemiologists. But it has been shown above that the special contribution of the general practitioner to the health team is diagnostic skill. In most other areas of practice his professional colleagues, whom he has brought in, are more skilled than he is. He should understand them without necessarily having their skills. The major source of physical diagnostic skill is still the hospital, so it must remain as one of the sheet-anchors of medical education. Greatly diminishing its contribution would almost certainly lead to the development of a different kind of doctor, even in general practice, and would diminish his value in the health teams based there. Moreover, of all the health professionals, it is only the doctor and the nurse who actually touch and manipulate patients' bodies. This is a most important relationship whose value to doctor and patient is frequently forgotten and misunderstood. It is an extra form of communication to be used for the benefit of the patient. Because of this, the rapport established between doctor and patient is of a different order from that of the other health professionals. It is not lightly to be cast away. The fact that much diagnosis is made on the history does not minimise this importance, for it is only the professional doctor's short-cut. The evidence from the history is firmly based on previous diagnostic knowledge derived from physical examination and comprehension of pathological and other diagnostic tests. They come essentially from hospital practice.

There is no doubt that hospital practice must be kept in perspective, so that it must not be over-emphasised in relation to general practice and public health, community medicine and epidemiology. These too are essential to understanding the Biology of Man. It may be regretted that prolonged exposure of students to hospital practice may distort their appreciation of proper relationships within medicine and the relationships of medicine with society. But the same is true of any professional discipline. All see the world through their own particular eyes, conditioned as they have been to select what is of importance to them, partly by education of the minds which inform them. If the basis of medicine is diagnostic skill, then there is no escape from this preliminary distortion at some point in education. Not everything can be done at the same time. Any distortion must be corrected later, though even this presupposes that we can recognise it, as if from some special superior vantage point, which is impossible, since each of us has a unique view of the world.

POSTGRADUATE EDUCATION

It has been proposed that the aim of undergraduate education is the production of a relatively undifferentiated doctor. The time for differentiation is after graduation. So far this has largely been a matter of individual choice. Not too long ago each new doctor could find himself welcomed into almost any branch of medicine. But in the developed Western world the values of the market-place now intrude. Not only does the graduate have to determine what interests him, he has to decide if what he wants to do is overcrowded with practitioners. In many specialties there is an apparent surplus of surgeons and physicians. And even the less glamorous specialties seem rapidly to be filling up. Society too has its say, since governments are now the largest employers of medical labour and by promulgating establishments for various specialties they, somewhat indirectly, determine the career choices of doctors. Nearly all governments are now attempting to push doctors into less desired specialties and they are trying to achieve what they believe to be a better distribution of medical manpower geographically, as between town and country and more and less attractive residential areas. Their campaigns have some limited success.

The response of the medical profession is what might have been predicted, dictated, as with other social groups, by self-preservation and replication. The doctors have decreased the time that they are prepared to devote to their medical tasks; they have increased the numbers of tests required to come to a diagnosis; they have multiplied the diplomas deemed necessary before a man can be counted a specialist and this takes him a longer time and has more sharply drawn the demarcation lines between one discipline and another. The increase in technical skills and erudition in the specialties has increased the need for teachers and examiners, both in charge of the replication process, and this process takes practitioners away from their tasks with patients, so that more practitioners are needed to fill the gaps in care. It is said that the quality of care for each patient thereby improves, and this explains why more and more doctors are needed to do what fewer did before. There is, of course, some truth in all this, though there remains an uneasy feeling that the process is also self-generating and may be going too far.

The aim of the nineteenth century and the early twentieth century was to produce an omnicompetent general practitioner at graduation. The splintering of medicine into more and more specialties has made this aim impracticable. This is the reason for shifting the aim of medical education to the production of an undifferentiated doctor at graduation. Thereafter he builds on his education in a restricted sphere to become a craftsman in one or two of them. But it is now realised that even this is not enough. The pace of advance in medicine is such that even the man who acquires a higher diploma in surgery or medicine or anything else is not a finished product. He must go on educating himself and he must be a perpetual student. By the better doctors this has been realised for some time but, as we have seen previously, when an idea gains sufficient weight of opinion behind it, there are moves for institutionalisation. This is now happening in that specialist registers are being compiled. In some cases it will be a condition of retention on the special register, and possibly even on the general register, that at various times the doctor shall undergo a course of further training. There is as yet no mention of examinations after these, but it will surely come. There is evidence here of the self-replication of the educators and examiners. It sometimes appears that medicine has become self-generating with fewer and fewer recurrences to its main basis in practice.

With a long history and so much criticism, much of which may be well founded, there are many calls for educational experiment. These are essentially designed to integrate the subjects which make up the Biology of Man. The Western Reserve University experiment in the u.s.a. in this field has been widely quoted and misquoted. Its intention was to take a medical topic and look at it from all relevant aspects, so that it was seen whole, for example in its physical, chemical, biological, psychological and social contexts. It was extremely interesting, especially whilst it retained the pristine enthusiasm of its originators. But there is no good evidence that it produced better doctors than any other system. The reason is not hard to find. It is because no one can properly define what a better doctor is, because his function in the community cannot be well defined, nor is medicine well defined, nor what society wants from it. Moreover, in different parts of the world, and even in different parts of the same country, different things are required of the doctor. And his character and knowledge and skills also have their effect in determining what is wanted from him.

One result of this enormous problem has been to retreat from it by trying to define a core curriculum. This seeks to answer the question 'What must every doctor know?' So far every attempt to give a satisfactory answer has failed, for again no one can agree on what is a standard doctor. A further retreat is then necessary to try to answer the questions such as 'What must every doctor know of anatomy, or physiology, or bio-chemistry or psychiatry?' Even this is almost a nonsense question for the same reasons as before, but gets a little nearer to what seems to be required. But it is inevitably subject to the pressures of the professionals in these various subjects, who over-estimate the importance of their subjects to the nebulous ideal doctor. The next phase becomes even more trivial in that it defines a small part of a subject which the teachers feel must be known. Because it is felt that education must become increasingly scientific a class is tested before the topic is taught; then it is taught, then the class is tested again to see how much of what has been imparted has been retained. It is trivial because it stresses teaching and its technology rather than learning and education. Yet more and more man-hours are being devoted to it year by year. It is remarkable that even students, bowing to authority, acquiesce in this process. Such is the anxiety generated to know exactly what they know and tick it off on a mythical list as known, that they have fallen victims to teaching rather than education. It reduces education to technology, taking away freshness, enthusiasm, adventure, excitement and personal exploration.

Medical pedagogues forever pay lip-service to motivation of students and how this may be achieved. It is well recognised that this is an emotional force, not an intellectual one. From this has arisen the call for the introduction of students to real medicine from their earliest years, which means the introduction of clinical medicine. The thought is that this will show the student the relevance of his studies in physics, chemistry and basic medical sciences to the patient and the future doctor's practice. It seems to contain an element of truth, but by no means for every student. The system of education in France does put students into the wards from their earliest days and does not seem to diminish the confusion of students in the learning of medicine. Neither did the system at Western Reserve. Motivation is essentially something arising from within and not imposed from without. Its reasons are immensely variable. It can receive a prod from an enthusiastic teacher but cannot be ingrained by him whatever the order of the course. Frequently it is the chance remark which revives the flagging motivation and not the consciously directed one.

The experimental method now extends to the conduct of examinations. They come in all sorts of shapes and sizes, and attempts are made to evaluate them. At least this serves the purpose of making examiners and teachers search their minds and hearts to try to determine what it is that they expect from examinations. At the postgraduate level this is relatively easy, for it is to some extent a testing of craft, and the examination cannot be reached without evidence of having served as an apprentice to some suitable master. But how is an examination to be conducted to tell if the candidate is educated? Or that he is suitable as a person to proceed from undifferentiation to differentiation? That this is so far an impossible question to answer is shown by the move from the all-embracing final examination to a series of assessments, either written or by *viva voce* or by simple old-fashioned opinion of the teachers. Now there are attempts to include assessments of students by their peers at various stages in the course. Again there is no good evidence yet that any one method is better than any other, and this stems again from the fact that to define what a doctor is and what he does, except in very strictly defined circumstances, is not possible.

There are aims of medical education, and there are objectives. These last are what particular teachers expect students to know of their particular subjects in a given time. They can be tested after a fashion. But education cannot, and yet it is the educated doctor that both the profession and society seem to want. Why they want educated, preferably wise men as doctors remains to be discussed. There is little doubt that much of present medical education is tending to squeeze out education and substitute instruction. It is not surprising since the essence of education is elusive, whilst the technological content of medicine is relatively easy to define. Fortunately the spirit of education is present in both teachers and students even though neither group can properly pin it down. If sought directly, rather like searching for happiness, it escapes. It is a by-product of the play of mind on mind and of experience. These are infinitely variable because they are individual.

Education is not achieved by curricula nor by examination. But both are still essential because medicine is an important arm of society, or at least society thinks that it is. Therefore society has a legitimate claim on the profession to see that its practitioners conform to some sort of standard. In general it may perhaps be fairly said that medicine has done this. It may not be the best standard attainable, nor may it be being achieved in the most economical way, but it has not so far seriously failed those whom it is designed to serve. The students and doctors who fall by the wayside and have failed the standards of medicine, as judged by their peers, are comparatively few, though this has the drawback for egalitarians that this is only an example of the medical profession judging itself. But this putting of power in medicine in the hands only of doctors is being remedied to some extent by the inclusion of nonmedical people on medical tribunals.

The future of medicine and its relationships with society are obviously partly in the hands of its younger members. They are developing the ethos of medicine just as the scientists of the past and present are developing the technology. Such young doctors and students are products of society just as much as they are of medicine. We have seen some of the response of medicine to the increasing numbers of doctors and the gradually diminishing availability of some jobs within medicine. It is the usual response of self-preservation and replication, even though these are largely unconscious. There is pressure for diminishing hours of work, for more leisure, for more time with families, for time to study and to take examinations for the furthering of their service to patients, who expect ever increasing standards of care. The result seems often to be a diminishing standard of care. It is probably technically more perfect, but humanly less so. Yet the general public, in a psychological age, asks for more human treatment, and judges medicine more by this than by technique. But the really personal doctor is a creature of the past except in the rarest instances. Patients are looked after by teams, whose personnel is constantly changing. They are seen in general practice and in hospitals. Some members of the team are never seen by the patient. They are in the background in diagnostic departments and laboratories. It is a fact of present-day medicine and society.

The less personal care probably means a change in attitude of the doctors to their place in society. It suggests that they see themselves as technologists rather more than as guides, mentors and friends and wise counsellors in the myriad vicissitudes of life. In this the craftsmen have overcome the educators, and may well give hostages to those who would see the doctor reduced in status in society and to those who would support 'trimming' his education. Their voices gain added strength by the attempts of the medical profession to keep their income well in advance of those of other professional groups. In an egalitarian age this is often resented, especially when it is thought that the reasons for these differentials in income are allied with a diminution in the kinds of service which the general public had been led to expect. If doctors are technologists and work no longer hours than anyone else it makes it increasingly difficult to maintain the image of a learned profession devoted only to the care of the sick. In this, as in so much else, the place of medicine within the scheme of things is changing rapidly. The essence of profession and of education, perhaps proceeding to wisdom, may be being lost. Some might welcome this and there is no doubt that the concepts of profession and education are nebulous. But these are probably the qualities that the public seek, and if they do not find them the repercussions for medicine and its practitioners may at least partially be foretold.

I I

Medicine the Commodity

If, by some remarkable agency, medicine was withdrawn from the earth, the majority of the world's population would not even know. They would not miss what they have never had. In 1966 the International Federation of Gynaecology and Obstetrics and International Confederation of Midwives published *Maternity Care in the World* (Oxford, Pergamon Press). In it they analysed births in different countries and the numbers of doctors and midwives available for help. The details are very interesting, but the main upshot was that in 95 per cent of the world's births there was no person with any professional knowledge of the process present, and every year there are about 90 million births. Similar studies in other disciplines of medicine would almost certainly show the same non-existent medical and nursing care. Estimates of population and of doctors are difficult to obtain with any accuracy, but this book gives the following numbers of doctors to population:

Africa   1 to 8,100
Americas   1 to   800, or 1 to 1,200, excluding the U.S.A.
Asia   1 to 2,600
Europe   1 to   800
Oceania   1 to 1,100
U.S.S.R.   1 to   600

So apart from Africa, Asia and much of South America the

number of doctors might seem to be reasonably satisfactory. But in fact their distribution leaves much to be desired. Doctors tend to congregate in the larger conurbations. They have a greater income there, they are among colleagues, and they have the resources of high-technology medicine to help them. In much of Africa there may only be one doctor for 50,000 of the people. There is no doubt of the uneven distribution of doctors. But it is not even possible to say how many doctors are needed for a given number of people. It all depends on the quality of care which is thought to be necessary and the resources which can be afforded and made available to the doctors to carry out their tasks.

People in capital cities and other large centres nearly all have access to therapeutic medicine at a price. The price is fixed by the doctors, by their fees and the resources they demand, in most areas, and it is determined more in relation to the status of the doctor and the level of income which he thinks he should have than in relation to the needs of the populace. This effectively limits most therapeutic medicine to the small section of the public which can pay for it. The remainder are relatively neglected, even though valiant efforts are often made to redress this imbalance by individual doctors, by government and missionary services. However, only in rare instances is it possible by these means to bring the best that medicine has to offer to anything but a small proportion of the public. In Britain it has largely been effected by the government controlling virtually all the health services and paying the doctors out of taxes. It was possible because the country as a whole was prosperous and could afford to pay about 5 per cent of its gross national product for health care. Other advanced countries could do the same, but in general have used various insurance methods to try to bring medical care to their peoples and distribute it fairly.

There is little doubt that entrepreneurial medicine, practised purely privately, in which the patient hires the doctor for a given illness, cannot evenly distribute medical care. Where insurance systems are operative the same is true. Care will be more evenly distributed than under purely private medicine, but there may be a large percentage of the population which cannot afford the insurance premiums. They then have to be cared for either by charity or government, or go without medical aid. In a developed democratic country it is more likely that medical care can be evenly distributed under a total government service than under either private or insurance systems. But democracy allows the doctors, in some measure, to decide where they will work and in what disciplines. Doctors cannot then be directed to unpopular geographical areas nor to unpopular disciplines, though incentives can be offered to attract them, and some minor disincentives can be applied to try to achieve a socially defined aim. Only dictatorships can achieve full medical coverage of their populations. Even they have their problems because of geographical isolation of some of their people. The conclusion must be that the really even distribution of all medical care is simply not possible, except at such high cost as to make it quite unrealistic. There will always be inequities, though some systems reduce these more than others.

A further consequence of the removal of medicine from developed countries, where its loss would be appreciated most, would be the large numbers of health workers thrown on to the labour market. Unemployment might rise alarmingly. In a complex society secondary, labour-intensive industries are valuable in keeping people occupied. The majority of workers are non-producers of goods and need to be employed in providing others with services. The need for these is self-generating, as with so much else in society, and where needs are not immediately evident they will be 'manufactured'. This process has been mentioned in connection with medicine; when the backlog of disease is overcome the expectations of the people are raised and more of what they would formerly have put up with is pulled under the aegis of medicine. But except at the very simplest levels there seem at present to be no other solutions than those of the expansionist society. The possible unpleasant consequences of this are seeping into thinking and have led to the calls for zero population growth, but the sequels to this are far from clear.

With zero population growth the age structure will change so that there will be an increasing number of middle-aged and older folk, living on the productivity of a relatively small number of the younger age-groups. Provided that there is an increased use of technology and greater invention this may continue to be possible. But if this does not happen there may well be a fall in the standard of living; food may become dearer and harder to get, whilst services such as water, gas and fuel supply may become harder to maintain. Moreover, it is probable that zero population growth will be achieved earlier in the developed and more highly educated communities than in poorer countries such as those of India and South America. This could result in rising populations in the poorer areas of the world at the same time as the developed countries were also becoming poorer and quite unable to help the backward. Of course the present economic system is such that even when there are surpluses of food in the developed countries there is no way to get it to the economically underprivileged. They cannot afford to pay for it, so it can only be given by the charity of the richer nations. But medicine, as at present organized, has very little part to play in these major economic problems. If it were withdrawn then more people would die of injury, of childbirth and of infections, and a few people might live less long and in greater discomfort than they otherwise might. On a full-blooded evolutionary biological view this would be right. It would be the proper extension of the notion of zero population growth.

Man is now brought sharply face-to-face with the fact of his biological nature. His exploitation of the environment has been so successful and his numbers are so vast that within limits the natural environment is subdued. The troublesome environment is himself, and the varying nations and groups struggle for their shares of what the environment, natural and man-made, has to offer. His success as a species has partly come about because of his psychological and social nature, one of the offsprings of which has been medicine. Medicine is counter-evolutionary.

In biological nature it is the species which is successful. The individual has little importance provided that individuals in the mass can remain at a certain critical level and continue to reproduce. The species needs a food supply, and capacities for self-preservation against predators, together with reproduction to keep up its numbers. The evidence suggests that the food supply of the species Man may be lagging behind requirements.

On the global scale there are now no predators which Man need fear. The only one likely to do him harm is his own species in war. The kind of war need not be military, it can be economic and financial. Against this biological background Man, in Western Christian societies, has set up a cultural ethos emphasising the importance of the individual, and an aspect of care for individuals is medicine. The choices begin to emerge with stark clarity. They are whether Man is to be envisaged as a species or as a collection of equally important individuals.

Pursuing his biological path *Homo sapiens* will continue on his expansionist way until he comes up sharply against himself as a major constraint. He seems to be getting near this point already. The Christian ethic has helped this biological expansion by making culture a handmaiden of biology. It has helped to care for individuals in food, housing, warmth, water supply, sewage disposal, communication and education. The species of Western Man has been very successful. He has managed to throw off some of the constraints of famine and disease, though wars continue to plague him. Although wars are fought with ferocity, they too are becoming increasingly matters of technology, so that the actual loss of life on the battle-fields is less than it used to be, so even this check on the species is not so very great. The great catastrophes of flood, fire, earthquakes and epidemics provide only limited checks too, for the birth-rate soon replaces those who perish.

These considerations put medicine in its context. The species of Man was being highly successful before medicine could have been of any real value in aiding him and abetting him. It is factors other than medicine which have been responsible for increasing birth-rates, lowering death-rates, controlling epidemics and increasing longevity. Medicine makes some contribution to these but it is very minor. It has much more to do with the quality of life than its quantity. It is not a necessity for Man; it is a gloss on his civilisation. It comes into its own when a particular society feels a need for it and becomes willing to provide the resources for it. And just as in the past when doctors were thinly spread and few could afford them and their services, so it still is with poorer societies and countries. Those who cannot afford the cost do without.

Medicine sprang from humanitarian impulses, bringing help to those in its own immediate circle, but it has always felt that it had an international flavour. Through its and many societies' evangelists it has tried to take medicine of some sort to every part of the world. To reduce suffering by medicine has become an article of faith. This is especially seen in the responses to death and destruction on a large scale, such as those of natural disasters and war. Those nations that can, rally round and fly in doctors, medical supplies, food and blankets. But when the major need is met, if only partially, the impulse to help fades away once more and the individuals in backward countries fall back onto meagre medical resources.

Suffering, disease and death are the lot of Man. They cannot be banished, they can only be minimised to some extent. Medicine is one of the agencies for this. But like everything else it cannot be brought in full measure to everyone. It is a commodity which some can afford and some cannot. Much as it may be desired, medicine is not everyone's right. The alternative for Man as a species can easily be borne, as it is at present in many parts of the world. Men, women and children suffer, fall ill and die. It is possible that those with access to medicine have less trouble with these individual disasters but that is by no means proven.

12

The Value of Medicine

Medicine is compounded of many things, so many that it can mean almost anything to anyone. It has been seen to grow from magic and the priesthood through the centuries until the days of modern science. On the way it received a large injection of the Christian ethic, and though it may no longer be overtly Christian the humanitarian ideal remains. At all times the development of medicine has been dependent upon the climate of opinion of the society within which it was practised. In particular it has always needed monetary support, and has thus been dependent upon local prosperity, and later on national commercial success. The evidence is clear that it has never been of primary importance to the earlier development of Man as a species, nor even to nations. They grew and became successful and increased their populations and economic and military power without any significant contribution from medicine. Medicine is only called into being on a large scale when the economic base of society is secure. This, of course, refers to curative medicine mainly. Preventive medicine has had rather large successes in helping the species, but engineers and technologists were at least as important in this, and a case can be made that the public works were well in hand and progressing before medicine annexed them to itself, especially through medical officers of local health authorities. It was only when they were able to explain the rationale of pure water supply, sewage disposal, clean food handling and so forth, after the rise of bacteriology, that preventive medicine became part of medicine at all.

Now preventive medicine has caught the governmental, medical and public eye. It can point to defects of all kinds in the environment, physical, mental, social and medical, and then social engineering can begin to make people healthier. There is disillusion with high-cost, high-technology medicine which deals with individuals one at a time. The lure of so changing the environment that fewer and fewer people will need this type of individual attention is exciting, and seems to have the merit that it will be less costly.

So the rainbow's end, the will o' the wisp, is chased again. Grandiose schemes are hatched. At first it was bigger and better hospitals, some laboratories, more research, and more and more teams specialising in erudite branches of curative medicine. The physical mechanism of Man could be put right like that of a motor car until the rust was so pervading that disintegration set in. But this has been seen not to increase health. It has, in fact, decreased it in terms of the numbers of people seeking medical care. But, as we have seen, this is largely because the definition of health has been constantly changing, and public and medical expectations of what constitutes health have risen. The change in emphasis to environmental medicine will not change anything. It will not make people healthier; it will only shift the scene of the action. Neither medicine nor anything else can take death, disease and suffering away from individuals and therefore the species. Perhaps it is time to acknowledge the fact and stop behaving as if these disasters could ever be banished. There is need to have realistic expectations both within medicine and society of what each can do for the other.

Medicine has no rights to expand in unlimited fashion, either in its research and technology, or in the numbers of doctors and the facilities they say they require. The arguments of medicine for these things are with society, which can put the limits where it wishes. These are usually placed by politicians acting as the voice of the public and dispensing their money gained through taxes. Doctors appeal to the humanitarian impulses of the people, and play upon their desires for relief, comfort and longevity, whilst the politicians dare not openly say that these cost too much in certain areas at certain times. Indeed, both sides to the argument are not candid either with themselves or the other side. This is probably largely subconscious and not cynical. They each believe what they say in humanitarian zeal, whilst they are, in fact, pursuing different aims from the ones they profess. Of course, each side does have humanitarian impulses, but one wants to conserve money to spend on other things than medicine, and medicine wants to preserve its high status within society.

There can be no full resolution of the 'dispute' between medicine and society. Like everything else in life medicine must continue with adjustments to its environment as this changes. There will be gains and successes as well as losses, seen from the viewpoint of medicine, and with some of the successes individual patients will have some relief and comfort that they might not otherwise have had. But in this shifting scene, who gets what will remain as arbitrary as it always has been. A life, or a disease and its relief, are not priceless. They are worth what society will pay for them one way or another. By virtue of many variable factors (the doctor, his team, his geographical location, his resources, and the patient and his disease) not everyone can have the best medical care at all times and in all places. This is true of the most developed countries and applies *a fortiori* to the underdeveloped ones. It is futile even to try to attain this perfect goal.

In pure accountancy terms, therefore, medicine can be seen as in some measure dispensable. As emphasised previously it is so dispensable that many parts of the world have had no access to it ever. And much of it could be dispensed with in advanced countries at a price for certain individuals of greater suffering than they otherwise might have had. It is fortunate for them that society has not yet taken a starkly realistic accountancy or evolutionary view of medicine. There is still more clinging to the humanitarian ideal, but it is being eroded in practice if not in overt thinking. Perhaps the main value of medicine is in the maintenance of public morale. This is what has been known to armies for a very long time; that the presence of the medical services gives confidence to the soldiers. It is right that humanitarian impulses and the boosting of morale should be given as much support as possible. They are apparently needed by all societies and should not be gainsaid in the worship of more mundane values. Medicine can give free rein to those within to indulge their altruistic qualities of helping, whilst preserving their *amour-propre*, and the public can see medicine as an arm of their concern, tenderness and mercy. This does not diminish medicine within society; it exalts it. Seen in this light there is no necessity for medicine to clamour for its place in the sun. It will for the foreseeable future have it, for society needs it, though not in the way that it has thought. The dangers to its position arise mainly from within, especially by misunderstanding of what medicine is and does for society. It is self-defeating to plead the high ideals of medicine, being in the forefront of society's desires for wanting to be seen displaying compassion, and at the same time by a variety of actions show only evidence of self-preservation and needless replication. The doctors have a place in society which is enviable. They can destroy it by exaggeration, unnecessary protest and a failure to understand themselves and the society within which they function.

13

The Future

The present places limitations on the future, which cannot be infinitely variable, at least in the short term. Change can only arise from the present base. Analysis of the bases gives some opportunity of deciding what the future may be. Previous knowledge of possible eventualities, derived from history, may make the analysis more secure. Nevertheless, the future must always remain uncertain because of unforeseen factors, and those to which a wrong weighting, in the event, have been given. However, the effort of trying to see what may happen can be worthwhile, for a selection might then be made from alternative courses. Choice becomes possible on a conscious basis. Foresight is one of the special attributes of Man, and should perhaps be employed. It is often a faulty instrument, but there is no better one for the purpose, and repeated attempts should be made to refine it. The future may be allowed to drift unconsciously into being, or it may be partially influenced by conscious selection from a number of possibilities. Which possibilities eventuate are determined by the prevailing climate of opinion, which can be influenced by persuasion. Fully rational choice of the future of medicine cannot be possible, because of the immensity of the subject and cultural emotional attitudes towards it, but more rather than less rationality may be used.

Since medicine has no separate validity from the society in which it is practised, it will continue to vary from place to place and especially from country to country. The cost of Western-type medicine is so great that only governments can now fund it, or arrange for its funding through some special scheme. The

nature of government, and its political philosophy, will determine the development of medicine in the areas within government control. Democracy will allow the doctors some voice, as
well as the people, whilst dictatorship may reduce the medical
contribution to determination of the future of medicine to any
level it wishes. The doctors in a dictatorship are employees of the
state and must do its bidding. In any partially literate community, having some contact with the outside world, there will
always be some medical care, even under a dictatorship.
Medicine is needed for morale and some internal cohesion, as
well as for the natural propensity of those in power to wish for
its aid when they fall ill. Some level of medicine is therefore
wanted, and if the country is rich enough, medicine will be
allowed some high-technology development, both for the
prestige of the country internationally and for the use of the
upper echelons of society when they need it. Russia and China
do this now, whilst the rich of Arabia and elsewhere buy the
services of Western medicine when they feel it is necessary.
They have to travel to the high-technology centres, because
their own human resources are not yet capable of this superior
level of medical achievement. The reason for this lies in poor
primary and secondary education, which cannot produce
students capable of taking advantage of tertiary medical
education on the Western model. Nor is the ethos of many Arab
and Far Eastern countries of a kind which puts high value on
individual lives of all members of their communities, so that
medicine may not be attractive as a career, or it is beyond the
means of students or governments.

In democracies the doctors still retain some powers of helping
to determine the direction of medicine. The medical profession
has for a long time had a very free rein in determining its own
destiny. It has favoured a continuation of eighteenth- and nine-
teenth-century systems of the delivery of medical care. Doctors
are individualists and in the main wish to be entrepreneurs.
They know that they have high skills, much sought after by
those who are ill, and they have high status. All rare goods and
services are expensive, so it has been possible for doctors to
command large fees, and their incomes have therefore been
towards the upper end of the range in virtually all recent com-

munities. However, medicine has not been only concerned with incomes and the medical profession. It has always had a very well developed social conscience and compassion. These are characteristics which have endeared the medical profession to the societies where it operates. There has been a selflessness and devotion to duty and work by many doctors, which has been immediately apparent, and has determined their high status. Society has commended the virtues of the profession, including the large element of charity, which doctors have often dispensed unstintingly. They have always been more aware of the unfortunate sufferers in society than any other comparable group of articulate educated people. It is because of this that so many philanthropists have arisen in their ranks, and they have pursued their goals for the benefit of other people – the poor, the sick, the old, and the underprivileged of all kinds. It has come to be expected that those forgotten by society will come to find a champion somewhere within medicine. Nobody is surprised when a doctor draws attention to an area of need. His status, moral and financial, and his fairness demand a hearing. He has often been the conscience of society and its eyes, because of his very special relationships with all sorts and conditions of men. It has for long been an enviable position of trust and integrity.

Because of its appeal to some of the best feelings within society, which give a glow of self-satisfaction, it has seemed right to extend the benefits of medicine more widely. This has meant increasing the number of doctors by expanding their production through medical education. It is a policy which has been wholeheartedly implemented in much of the Western world. The morality, the essential rightness of medicine, could not be called into question. If ten times as many doctors could be called into being, so the argument seemed to run, there would be a tenfold increase of caring within society, and that could not be other than right. The motives were surely unexceptionable. So more and more doctors have been produced.

More doctors, however, have not procured the apparently desired results. The ultimate reasons for wanting them were not defined. The unspoken expectations were, perhaps, that more doctors would give more care, demonstrate more concern, save more lives, and bring more relief, more comfort and more longevity to the communities in which they worked. It may be that all these things have happened, but it is not immediately apparent. If both society and medicine had stayed still, then more doctors would almost certainly have done what was wanted. But both have changed, so that firm baselines for comparison cannot be established. Without them it is not possible to be sure whether the objectives have been certainly achieved.

Medicine has become technically more complex. Disease patterns have changed, but not so greatly in some parts of the world as in others. Therefore the aims and objectives of the medical services must vary according to geography. The sorts of doctor recruited to the different services must therefore differ. Except in the very broadest terms medicine is not truly international. In the highest reaches of technical attainment it may be, but in the delivery of medical care it is not. It may be possible to cross the national boundaries in talking of patients as physical beings, but their psychology, psychiatry and social organisations make cross-cultural understanding almost meaningless. The difficulties are made greater by language barriers. There can be an international communication of value only within scientific medicine. The Western-type doctor, however great his numbers, cannot seriously contribute to the delivery of medical care to communities culturally different from his own. Health care delivery is so dependent upon cultural acceptability that there will be few outlets in underdeveloped countries for Western doctors.

With modern concepts, therefore, medicine has become parochial. It has tried to consider its benefits as universally applicable, and should now realise that they are not. Doctors must be produced by and for their own cultures. There is not a universal doctor, though there can be a universal super-specialist in some branch of medicine, provided that he works only at the physical level as a technologist. This kind of person can work anywhere if he is given the appropriate resources for his techniques, but even these may not be forthcoming because of their cost. Moreover, this medical technology requires teams of people, and the educational system of a particular country may not be able to produce them at a sufficient degree of attainment.

It seems, therefore, that doctors will remain, as they always have done, within their own cultures. There are few outlets for their skills elsewhere. It is fortunate for English-speaking doctors that the British culture has spread so far and wide. It still embraces:

Canada	21,568,000	population	(1971)
U.S.A.	203,212,000	population	(1970)
Australia	12,728,000	population	(1971)
New Zealand	2,863,000	population	(1971)
U.K.	55,522,000	population	(1971)
Total	295,893,000		

which is about 8%–9% of the world's population. It perhaps needs no arguing that the British culture is in some measure of retreat in places like Africa, India, Singapore, Hong Kong and elsewhere where it once held sway.

The number of doctors in the above areas are about:

Canada	20,000	Dr to population ratio	1:1,078
U.S.A.	245,000	Dr to population ratio	1: 829
Australia	16,100	Dr to population ratio	1: 790
New Zealand	3,500	Dr to population ratio	1: 818
U.K.	62,000	Dr to population ratio	1: 895

The figures are all very approximate.

There is, of course, a well-known influx of Western-type doctors in all these cultural areas, from India and many other underdeveloped areas. Again, this seems likely to be diminished by political action in the poorer doctor-producing countries.

Many advanced nations seem to have reached a doctor-population ratio of about 1 to 800. This seems to provide enough doctors to support primary care or general practice in the community, and secondary care in hospitals, together with a fair provision of what have come to be known as super-specialties. These include neurosurgery, cardio-thoracic and vascular surgery, radiotherapy and other cancer services. It is probably a reasonably generous staffing ratio for the provision of high-quality medical care. However, it does not cover all medical care in all places at all times. There is uneven distribution of doctors between the specialties, as well as between primary, secondary and tertiary care, and also between urban and rural areas, and between different parts of cities. It is a dream of planners to iron out these disparities in the accessibility of all people at risk to appropriate medical care. This is not possible either in a dictatorship or a democracy. Certain low-level services can be given to remoter rural areas with scattered populations by coercion of doctors in a dictatorship or by persuasion of various kinds in a democracy. But provision of high-cost care to all is unproductive and cannot be achieved under any political system. It could only be done with infinite resources, and a willingness to waste human, financial and technical skills. The next best thing is to build up centres of ever-increasing complexity from the periphery to the hub of concentrated technical expertise. This is what is being done, so that all the people can have reasonably easy access to simpler medical care and, as they need it, they can be transported to places of greater skills. This is the theory. In practice there can be human failures, especially in peripheral doctors not recognising the limitations on their own capabilities, so that they undertake too much of matters beyond their competence. However, it is doubtful if any better form of organisation can be developed. It therefore remains only to make it more efficient.

Improving medical efficiency almost inevitably involves some form of audit. The evolution of the doctor so far in the Western world has made this concept unwelcome to the medical profession. The fiction has been maintained that all doctors are equally competent in clinical situations, when manifestly they are not. It has been assumed that all doctors will always do their best and will always be up-to-date and competent. This is a remnant of thinking from the nineteenth century when a good doctor probably could encompass the known science of medicine. Now he cannot, so he has to discover for himself where his knowledge is inadequate for his tasks. Some can do this on their own, but they are few. Already in many branches of medicine audit is accepted and it is being practised. It takes the form of review of cases and critical assessment of what was done for each patient, what was the outcome, whether good standards of practice were maintained, and whether something better might have been achieved. A whole group of doctors can in this way formally learn from each other and so improve practice. As with so many other areas of group behaviour, this one will spread and almost certainly will become institutionalised.

A further step along the road of checking on the doctors will be to test their knowledge of their subjects at intervals through their professional lives. Audit is a form of continuous personal assessment. Thereafter may come external assessment by peers. To make this effective will need some form of sanction against those who do not reach the required standard. The only one is removal from the general or specialist medical register or the requirement of a special course of further training to allow of the retention of a name on the register. Since the register is maintained by, or is under the aegis of, a governmental agency, this testing of doctors' competence will become statutory. Politics and society will have encroached further on the autonomy of medicine. The medical profession will have begun the process, which will ultimately be taken largely out of their hands. They will administer the scheme since no one else can, but they will do it as agents for society, and not as their own masters.

The use of external audit, probably by examination of some kind, raises the old dilemma of what exactly is to be tested and assessed. What does the doctor do, and what is medicine? For the specialist the answer is fairly easy. There is normally a recognised body of knowledge in each subject. It is within the keeping of the various Royal Colleges, or their faculties. The knowledge required of such specialists is largely of a technical nature. The material of practice is far less clear for general physicians, general surgeons and general practitioners. They try to keep a competence over a wide field, though this is diminishing rapidly. In the larger conurbations, where major hospitals can be supported, the specialties have so encroached on general medicine and general surgery, that these subjects are now scarcely recognisable. The general practitioner normally channels his patients to specialists, when they are needed. General physicians and general surgeons are only required when a full range of specialist services cannot be provided. This occurs when a population served is too sparse, geographically isolated and perhaps widespread. Services supporting such general physicians and surgeons, such as radiology and pathology, are also conducted at a less efficient level than is attainable with a high volume of work in a metropolis. The further from the major centre the less the technical excellence will usually be. The standards at the periphery must be lower than at the centre because of lack of resources – human, technical, financial, and in building. This fact is already tacitly recognised by medical planners and allocators of money. High-level technical skill cannot be made available to everyone wherever he may be. Good rapid transport to a major centre can only be a partial substitute for the lack of local resources and expertise. In this sense, life, relief, comfort and longevity are deemed less important for peripheral populations than central ones. It is likely always to remain so. There are limits to what can and what will be provided.

Not only are physical resources less freely available peripherally, but also the professional isolation normally reduces the knowledge and skills of the health personnel. This can only be partly offset by refresher courses, travelling lecturers, audio-visual aids, television programmes, journals, and other educational devices. They are no full substitute for the day-to-day contact of experts solving problems together and sharpening mind on mind.

In terms of medical technique, specialisation improves patient care. It may be argued that this may diminish the understanding and the needs of the patient because he is removed from his psycho-social environment, isolated in hospital and has attention concentrated only on one organ or system which is supposedly physically deranged. This can happen, but often is an exaggeration. Not always is the psycho-social environment of importance, a fact most obviously observed in an acute medical or surgical emergency, though the whole person again assumes significance during convalescence. At an opposite pole many neuroses and some psychoses are mainly dependent on the psycho-social environment for their causes, treatment and prognosis. The contribution of all factors in a patient's illness must ideally be assessed for diagnosis and management. There may be a tendency for the specialist to over-emphasise the factors which he understands best, but equally the generalist may under-estimate factors which he does not fully comprehend. There is no monopoly of wisdom in either. It is appreciation of this which has led to medical care being provided by teams of doctors and their allied health professionals, rather than by single-handed practitioners assuming a mantle of omnicompetence. This type of doctor is an anachronism in developed societies. But in poorer societies there is increasingly a willingness to accept something less than the best possible with unlimited resources, and have 'barefoot doctors', as in China, delivering at least some care.

There is a spectrum of medical care running from groups of super-specialists in major metropolitan hospitals through general physicians and surgeons, especially in smaller peripheral hospitals, general or family practitioners to the barefoot doctors, to no care at all of any professional kind. This kind of organisation will persist, though with local modifications, movements of groups and alterations of their functions within the system. Choices, conscious or unconscious, can be made about developments to be made at either end of the spectrum. The central part of it is unlikely to change very much. It has evolved historically and has come to be accepted as a part of Western culture, but this emphasises that it does not have to be part of every culture, as so many Westerners appear to believe.

Family practitioners have now developed teams of health-care professionals to help them in their tasks. The first point of contact of the patient (or client) with the health services is often now not a doctor, but someone less educated and trained in medicine. Frequently it is a nurse or pharmacist. In remote areas, and where doctors' fees are high, this has always been so, but it is being adopted as a deliberate policy, both by doctors and governments. Doctors are becoming more inaccessible again. Once they were inaccessible because many patients could not pay their fees. Now, even if government or some other agency pays the doctor's fees or salary, he tends to become more remote from his patient because of the team which surrounds him. The myth of the wise, kindly, instantly available family doctor has never been sustainable, except in a most restricted way, for this is a middle-class image. With really open access of all to the doctor he usually cannot cope on his own and requires his team, and this demonstrates that much of the dis-ease presenting to the family doctor is deemed by him to be not medical, but something else. There is again the dilemma of deciding what is medical and what is not. Some would include almost everything human, and others would exclude much that is psycho-social. The present trend is to expand the scope of medicine in the community, both in extending care to all and by accepting the wider categories of dis-ease. The choice of expansion or relative contraction of family practice is made mainly by individual doctors, or groups of them working together. The reason for their choice is usually one of temperament, an unconscious assessment that one form of practice rather than another suits the personalities of the doctors concerned. The rejection of some part of practice and acceptance of some other part has always been a matter for each doctor to decide. It has the merit that each is most likely to practise those parts of medicine at which he is expert, because of his interest.

The expansion of medical care in the community receives moral and financial support from government. The policy shows them as caring and concerned for their people and may allay some criticisms. The major ones are that hospitals have taken far too much of the resources made available for health, and that patients should be looked after in their own environments. On the face of it this form of practice in the community seems to have the merit of being cheaper than providing custodial care of whatever kind, and this has attractions, but the capacity for extending community care is limitless, so that, as with hospital care, decisions will be made about the extent of resources which will be allowed, and, in fact, family practice too will have limits placed on it.

In hospitals also there is a tendency to expand various forms of medical care, which usually arise out of scientific and technical advances. There is a natural desire for hospitals to wish to be in the van of progress and to use new techniques and instruments. But much of such progress is trivial, in the sense that benefits may be slight, if any, for individual sufferers, or alternatively any benefit may only accrue at high cost. This is especially exemplified in renal and cardiac transplantation. These show the ultimate results of pursuing the philosophy that virtually every life is worth saving, whatever the cost to the community. It is now apparent in practice that this view, despite its immense general emotional appeal, is no longer stoutly maintained. Value judgements have to be made about individual lives, the criteria for these being far from clear and liable to vary as much as the people who make them. There is a creeping acceptance of the Darwinian view of the evolutionary importance of the species as against the individuals of which it is composed, and a recognition that this probably applies to Man too. By the resources made available in different areas there is tacit consent that not all lives at all times and in all places are equally important and valuable. This basis for medical practice is not possible because to carry it fully into effect is far beyond the resources ever likely to be available. Yet much of Western medicine is being emotionally based in the belief that all must have an attempt made for them to have equal comfort and length of life. It is the ground for appeals for money for increasing research, for building health centres and hospitals, for buying new equipment, in short for expansion. Much heat is generated when these appeals are denied, and it is then said that for lack of money, lives are being needlessly wasted. Emotion and long conditioning put almost limitless value on an individual life; reason and practicality reduce its worth severely according to time and place, and circumstance. With the diminishing hold of religion, it is the community which tacitly allots value to lives by the resources it makes available through medicine to its members. Society claims to hold to an ideal view, which it pretends to try to bring to fruition, but which in practice it cannot fulfil, and it is likely that it never will be able to. There is a lack of realism both in society and in medicine.

Lack of realism extends to medical research and medical education. A vast amount of research is conducted in universities, research institutes and pharmaceutical companies. Most of it is unproductive of anything of immediate practical application for the benefit of patients. Even when something worthwhile is discovered it is slow to come into operation. This is because most research is scientific and technological and can only be adopted and used at this level, mainly in hospitals, where this kind of expertise resides. For a piece of fundamental research to be put into action it has to be accepted by practitioners who recognise its significance for them and for their patients, and these doctors must also have the resources to be able to use the new knowledge. There is thus inbuilt delay in appropriate practitioners hearing of the new work, accepting it and obtaining the facilities they need. Moreover, fundamental research is not often conclusive, so that its application in clinical practice may have results quite different from those expected. Thus, further research is often needed to be able to move from fundamental work to its application. But most research does not lead to practical application; only to accumulation of knowledge and understanding. That, however, is the main object of research for the researcher. His chances of making a really fundamental discovery are slight, but in his research he will be satisfying his own curiosity, modifying his own ideas and helping to change attitudes to old problems. It is this last which is perhaps the most important outcome of research, which is a practical manifestation of people testing and re-testing old and new ideas. This explains why most research appears practically unproductive at first sight, when looked at too narrowly. Benefactors of medical research must often be disappointed in the practical results of the financial investment that they make. They would like to have a 'cure for cancer', but instead they find their money has added only a little piece of knowledge not of immediate use. The research effort in medicine is evidence of medical society thinking and exploring for new hypotheses. These, which are often inexplicit, determine practice, and therefore can be very important for patients. It is suggested that the hypotheses and the climate of opinion out of which they arise and which they also help to generate are more important than the research itself. Ideas are more transmissible than results. Yet the practicalities of research are important in order to prevent hypotheses from becoming sheer idle speculation.

Realism suggests that a great deal of research masquerades as solving practical problems, when in fact it is about changing opinions, and trying to win over to those opinions an increasing number of people. When such a new opinion prevails it will be carried into practice, and may then become an accepted canon of medicine. Research then is essentially about thinking and persuasion. If this is realised and accepted, better value judgements could be made about individual researches. The question would be asked whether the underlying thought was valuable or not, and whether the projected work's outcome would be persuasive.

Research by those who are essentially teachers, though it may be of practical application, is mainly done for their own benefit, so that they may be testing their thinking and attitudes. This preserves freshness and enthusiasm and the exploration of ideas, which are perhaps the qualities which should best be imparted to their pupils. Most university research is of this nature. Its justification lies in the value which society at large is prepared to put on medicine and the education in universities for its practice. If society changes its judgement of the worth of medicine, and decides that the present attitudes towards the importance of each life, and its comfort, must diminish in intensity, then not all medical research and medical education can be deemed worthwhile, and their rate of expansion, as at present, is not a foregone conclusion. In fact there are already some signs that society is beginning to call for some contraction both of research and education. The body of medicine finds this unpalatable, but there is little point in raising too vociferous an outcry, for society, one way or another, is the final arbiter. It provides the resources and defines the aims, and medicine is only one of many claimants on society. In an age of expansion, medicine too can expand, and in an age of contraction, medicine must contract. It has no independent validity.

The value judgements about medicine, on which so much of the future of Western medicine depends, are contributed to by the public image of the medical profession. Formerly this has been one of a devoted, caring, self-sacrificing, somewhat unworldly group of people, dedicated to their work for the suffering and dis-eased. But the doctors are not separate from society, and they are affected by its values. These have been adopted by the profession so that now it is coming to be seen as no worse and no better than any other group of comparable education and training. The rigours of these, and the idea that a professional agent must be highly rewarded to guarantee that he will pay full attention to one's problems, have kept the doctors on high incomes. Moreover, these compensated for some of the doctor's adverse working conditions, in terms of hours on duty and residence required within easy reach of patients. By clamour for these conditions to be ameliorated, a process which is being continued and put right, the profession has discarded its claim to special consideration and attention. Its status has diminished, and this has called into question compensation at a high level for problems and difficulties which no longer exist. Status cannot be maintained when its base has been eroded. This can be seen in the rise and decline of the clerics over the last few centuries, and the high status of the doctor belongs only to the last 150 years or so. Before that time the vast majority of the doctors, surgeons and apothecaries were deemed little above the level of tradesmen. There is now diminishing reason for the public to consider the medical profession as having special merits, not possessed by others. This gains added force if there is a relative over-production of doctors. Elitism then has no claims. The labour market becomes depressed. Moreover, the doctors trim the corpus of medicine by handing over some of their former tasks to other health professions, thus making fewer medical men necessary.

Medicine could be in decline, despite some immediate evidence of expansion. Decline, in this context, means a diminishing value to society. It never has had high value in many, indeed most, parts of the world. It has recently, mainly because of technical achievement, attained high esteem, but this achievement has become counter-productive for society. It devours resources and has not fulfilled many expectations. Medicine has a place in society, but it is not as great a one as many have thought. Its value is being more narrowly defined than formerly and its potential is now recognised as finite.

Questions spring readily to mind:

How international is medicine?
It is international at a physical level, but not at the psycho-
social. A recipient under-developed country has to decide the
place of technological medicine within its own system, largely
as back-up to whatever primary-care services it has been able
to build. When these are known, more developed countries
which may well be producing more doctors than they need
might be persuaded to pay for them to work in the more backward areas. If there is real concern for all the world's population
the richer countries will not seek recompense for the medical
services they provide to those poorer than themselves.

*Should there be 'substandard' doctors? If so where, and what sorts of
people should they be?*
'Substandard' doctors are essential, because doctors are too
expensive and take too long to educate and train. Less than full
medical care has always been with us. Even in advanced
societies the nurse and the pharmacist often fulfil this role.
When there is no practical hope of providing doctors to look
after people it is essential to get 'barefoot doctors' of a kind
suitable for a particular community. Even in developed countries there is a place for such health workers, in remote areas
which are sparsely populated and where doctors cannot be
attracted. Often a nurse takes on these duties, but if he or she
is to take on responsibility for primary care, special training over
a short period would seem to be best, both for the nurse and
the community served.

*What is medicine in the community for? Why are we expanding it? Why
are we building up health teams?*
Essentially all health care is about relief, comfort and longevity.
People want these things, and doctors want to give them, as far
as is within their power, which derives from what individuals
and society will give for those benefits.

The expansion of medicine in the community comes about
because of the belief that it is not possible to have too much of
a good thing. This needs serious reappraisal, for carried to
extremes it becomes nonsense. Absolute relief, comfort and
longevity can never be had, so the questions arising are how

much of them do you want? and how much are you prepared to pay? When these are answered, the limits on expansion are clear.

The building up of health teams is based on the above belief, and on definitions of disease, which constantly raise expectations that cannot be satisfied. Moreover people have trained themselves to belong to expanding health teams, and specialism has increased, so that if there is no job for them to slip into, it becomes important, for economic and status reasons, to manufacture an area of need. Attitudes must change to make expectations realisable.

What is the importance of high-technology medicine?

It is very important to individual patients, but in terms of species-based medicine it is not important at all. It has as its fundamental thought that each person's life is valuable and should be fought for to the limit. In practice, of course, there is some falling away from this ideal. Another important consideration is the interest in high technology of those who practise it. There is immense satisfaction for them, at all levels of health care, in being helpful and useful to certain patients, whilst also facing intellectual and scientific challenges. In this way high-technology medicine is as important as any other human activity carried on at the limits of knowledge. Being in this field and contributing to it is as important to its participants as the climbing of mountains is to mountaineers, or the discovery of new things about the universe is to astronomers. This motivation is neither better nor worse than that displayed in most other human endeavours, which are thought by society to be valuable. But because of the purpose of high-technology medicine, often thought to be that of saving lives, it has greater emotional appeal than many other activities. It is therefore a value judgement as to how much of society's resources should be put into high medical technology as distinct from other areas of importance to society at a given time and place. At present the judgement seems to be that the rate of growth of high technology should be slowed, whilst that, say, of community care should be stimulated. Neither judgement of worth is of necessity either right or wrong.

What is the desirable number of doctors in different communities? How are they to be educated and for what functions?

As before this is a matter of judgement. It depends on aims. The 'fault' in the past is that these have not been specifically stated. Those responsible for decisions about the number of doctors needed have made unrealistic assumptions about the purposes of medicine, and have further assumed that what they believe is accepted by others. For the future, therefore, reasonable long-term aims must be agreed, and then objectives can be realistically determined. Such objectives, to be attained over a definite time, require foreknowledge of resources, particularly finance, which can be counted upon. This is the importance of the Health Commission to be considered later, to which body firm allocations should be given by government.

It is probable that the present ratio of doctors to populations in Western societies is about right for the time being, and there should not be automatic expansion based on emotional appeals. If Western countries are to expand the production of doctors it should be for limited objectives, which might for the moment be defined in terms of limitation of high technology, stimulation of community care and a policy for giving medical care, of limited type, to under-developed countries.

The education of doctors should remain an education and not a training for specific functions. Nurses, physiotherapists, pharmacists, psychologists, radiographers, laboratory technicians and 'barefoot doctors', as well as many others, can be trained to do a definite job. This can immediately determine their curricula, which deal with the present and the foreseeable short-term future. Training can, for them, be quite quick, and trainees can be useful at graduation. But society, and medicine also, need generalists, who cover a wide range of disciplines so that they may be adaptable to the long term needs of society, and the generalists may help to determine those needs. There is thus training for the present, and education for the longer term. Of course, there is education within training, and training within education, but it is possible to discern differences in function of the 'specialists' and the 'generalists'. Biological evolution shows the danger to the species when specialisation of function is overtaken by environmental change. The same can be seen in psycho-social evolution, with social changes making certain trades and industries superfluous. When this happens, it is those retaining the power of adaptation to the new circumstances who survive. This is not an argument simply for the survival of doctors. It is instead an argument that medicine should be responsive to the changing needs and judgements of society and be able to put them into action.

The wide base of present medical education should not, therefore, be narrowed, though there is a case for removing much of the curriculum, which is the accumulated deadwood of history, and perhaps for adding other subjects. But any new curriculum should not be built on any idea of producing a doctor for certain specific present needs, for they will certainly change in the future. The aims should be to preserve and enhance the adaptability of medicine as a whole, whilst accepting the fact that not all individual doctors will have that adaptability.

After the education of the undergraduate period must come the more craft-orientated postgraduate years of study. These can be too narrowing and need constant critical appraisal to make them retain a large part of the generalist concept. There is a tendency for the increasingly specialised to make their disciplines more esoteric. Constant efforts must rather be made to make specialisation and its methods simpler, so that they may be taken into the armamentarium of the more generalised. The erudite can usually do this, because they do not need to develop a priesthood, which is the keeper of the keys. It is the weaker ones who need the security of their special disciplines and who hedge it round with unnecessary difficulty.

How far should medicine be involved in population control?
If society is involved in this, then medicine is also. Medicine is not for itself alone, it is for society and is a response to its needs, whether these are emotionally or rationally based. This does not gainsay the fact that individual doctors, at least in a democracy, may not wish to engage in this control, but there are many other medical activities where they can fill a proper role in society.

What aspects of human existence should be shed from the canon of medicine?
Probably none. Historically, medicine has, through many of its practitioners, become involved in most human activity. This impetus cannot now be braked, and if doctors are truly educated as advocated previously, then society will benefit through medicine as a whole displaying interest in all human affairs.

What limits are being placed on medicine by society? Are they reasonable? How far should medicine resist these limitations?
The limits which society places on medicine are those of the resources which it will make available, and these and their extent arise out of nebulously held ideas about the place and value of medicine within society. Therefore the limits are reasonable by reference to the inadequately delineated climate of opinion. But medicine has been just as remiss as society at large in the definition of its place in society. It is this which it must make clear, so that suitable judgements can be made.

It is proper that medicine should resist the limitations which society imposes upon its activities. This is the right and duty of every subsociety. But medicine should be articulate, intelligent and analytical about itself. It has the capacity and intellect to be so. If it will use these characteristics and turn them to some purpose it will carry on a continuous dialogue with the various societies from which it derives and for which it was called into being. And this medicine will always need to do and go on doing, since societies are forever changing in time and in place.

14

Trial Solutions?

The previous arguments suggest that it may be idle to try to produce a blueprint for the better organisation of medicine in the future. It is probably best to take the Popperian solution, which has been put into a formula:

$$P_1 \longrightarrow TS \longrightarrow EE \longrightarrow P_2$$

This means that there is a first problem (P_1). It is vital that this be analysed in the most critical terms possible. But this will never be a full definition, for it is in the nature of human analysis that always something of importance, which will seriously affect the outcome of the solutions to the problem, is left out and not foreseen. So TS is the trial solution of the problem. It is not to be expected that it will be the final solution, because of those factors which were unforeseen. When it becomes obvious where the trial solution is failing, the next step is Error Elimination, which means the correction, as far as possible, of the undesirable side-effects of the trial solution. But these corrections alter the nature of the original problem, so that a second problem (P_2) arises. Again further analysis is required so there has to be another TS and another EE and then another problem. There is no finality in solutions and it should not be looked for. The dynamic nature of life has already been emphasised sufficiently. It is a matter of process and adjustment without ending.

'Does the road wind uphill all the way?
    Yes, to the very end.

Will the day's journey take the whole long day?
From morn to night, my friend.'
D. G. Rossetti

A major element in producing a plan for the future of medicine in society is the relationship of medicine to particular societies at the moment. It has been made plain that medicine is not the same in the different societies in which it is practised. And just as there is relativity between societies in space, so there is relativity in time, not all societies being at the same stages of development. The advanced societies are truly exploring, since they can have no maps to guide them in their quest for the proper place of medicine in society. But the poorer under-developed societies do have the example of developed medicine in front of them, so that they can choose whether to follow that pattern or not.

In fact, the really poor societies have few choices, because of the lack of resources needed to introduce Western-type medicine. They may be able to build hospitals, and even be able to put some high technology equipment into them. But in the foreseeable future they will be quite unable to produce Western-type doctors, who have a long course of undergraduate and postgraduate training and education, in sufficient numbers to serve their populations. They have to keep in mind that present Western medicine seems to require something of the order of one doctor to 800 of the population. They need progress in other fields rather than in medicine. These include food production, birth control, sewerage, water supply, housing and education, which are probably much more important for the real health of these societies than medicine. There are signs that this is being realised by many governments. If there is concern for the welfare of the populace then these other public health interests will come before medicine. And the process will be slow. Western medicine has taken something like 300 to 350 years to reach its present state, and it has done it only against the background of other developments within its own society. Under-developed countries will have to go through some similar sort of process, and it cannot be compressed into five- or ten-year programmes. There is, however, little doubt that the process can be compressed and made more rational, for developing societies can learn from previous experience of the West and adapt at least some of Western medical and public health technology to their own needs. Perhaps the right approach for an under-developed country is not even to try to imitate curative Western medicine at all, but simply to let its own kinds of health care develop as they will. This would mean that individuals would have to pay for their own medical care, if they wanted it at high technology level, whilst those who could not afford it would be dependent upon charitable impulse and the minimum type of health care which the country could afford, probably of a 'barefoot doctor' type. The really rich and the ruling classes could purchase their personal medical care from outside their country of domicile. This is happening now, and perhaps there should be little attempt to try to reverse it. The alternative, if it were possible, might be suddenly to introduce the whole gamut of Western medicine into the community, and the result would probably be disastrous. Public health measures might increase longevity, and with this would come a rise in population, which could not be fed and for whom jobs could not be found, whilst the health services might run away with an unacceptable proportion of the gross national product. The goals for medicine in an under-developed society must be kept realistic and that means that acceptance of relief, comfort, and longevity for all is not an immediately attainable objective.

Although charity begins at home, and is manifestly seen to do so in Western countries, an alternative solution for under-developed countries would be for developed countries to supply to the less well-endowed some health care from their own resources. Again, there are signs that this is being done, but it is on such a small scale that it cannot bring medical care of Western standards to all those deemed to need it. This means that since medicine grows out of the economic background of its own society, and since it will not in the foreseeable future grow out of its indigenous under-developed society, the West should supply the medical care from its own resources, and not expect payment from the recipient country. Western countries might then appear to be acting as did the missionary societies of old. Attention has already been drawn to some of the comparisons between the institutions of the church and of medicine. If medicine is an article of faith, as in some senses it is, then it may not be too fanciful to consider exporting it, not as a commodity to be bought, but as a charity to be dispensed. This would need profound alterations in thought by Western society, and particularly within the sub-societies of doctors. Nations, like individuals, find it hard to give to charity things which are other than superfluous to their felt needs. The sacrifice might be too great. Recipients of charity also often find it hard to accept. But if there should come an over-production of doctors in Western nations, which seems at least possible, then a solution such as export of doctors might become more feasible.

In Britain and Australia a policy of increasing the output of doctors has been and is being put into effect. The present doctor : patient ratio is about 1 : 800. Over the next twenty years it may fall to 1 : 400. There has never been any decision on what the upper limit should be. The figures have come about without any plan being thought out, but it seems to have happened as a result of trying to improve health by making medical care more available to everyone. But, as we have seen, the response of the doctors has been to diminish their hours of work, to have more leisure, to seek out pre-symptomatic disorder, to increase the scope of community practice, and to increase research and technology, all of which demand ever-increasing numbers of doctors. At the same time medical incomes have remained high so that fees and salaries have risen in an attempt to preserve the place of the doctor in society. Something similar seems to have been occurring in medicine in North America. Such responses are like those of trade unions whose interests appear to them to be threatened. Society in these Western countries seems not to have found any answer to the demands made upon them by their various sub-societies. Both in Britain and Australia the response has been to succumb to the demands, rather than forgo the benefits which these sub-societies contribute to the general welfare. However, there are retrenchments in various industries as consumer resistance builds up. It is happening in transport, mining, and the docks as well as elsewhere. Efforts to cushion the blows to workers in these and other industries are made by governments, on the basis of their not very explicit philosophies, but when society shifts its favours under economic impact, industries wither. The alternative of going without a commodity or service becomes preferable to paying too high a price for it. Those who supply the goods or services then suffer.

These general responses of society begin to be apparent in medicine. Individuals find that they cannot afford to pay for medical care delivered by private practitioners. They still want medical care, so the load is spread between individuals by insurance schemes. In time, even these costs begin to be too much for many people. The government then steps in to pay for much of medical care out of taxes. There later comes little alternative to providing medical care by salaried doctors. The salaries are then under government control and the price of medicine can be made to fit the pocket of the consumer. And it is medicine, and its practitioners, who bring this about. Their kind of pressure upon society always brings about the same response. Although the National Health Service in Britain started out in 1946 with different aims, this is the position now. The introduction of Medibank in Australia is part of a similar process. Society seems to have found the means for controlling medicine and its supply, whilst still groping for the means to control other sub-societies, largely represented by trade unions. At the same time, of course, society still puts a high value on medicine and so is willing to pay a high price, though not an exorbitant one, for it.

There are often political moves, as in Britain now, inspired by theoretical socialism, to try to get rid of private practice in medicine, or at least to make private practice difficult to pursue. However, private medicine should still continue, partly because many patients want it and so do many doctors. More-over, those who do private practice are seen by those who do not do it, but who work for the government either directly or indirectly, as guarantors of some liberty for the medical pro-fession. They are a symbol of importance. As long as private practitioners exist there is a half-formed thought in the rest that they too could opt out of the governmental system, or alter-natively increase their bargaining power with the government by threatening to do so. Since, regrettably, governments do not have a very good record as employers, it is not surprising that a weapon in the hands of the medical profession will not lightly be thrown away. It is probably wiser not to try to coerce them to do so, since it is now almost inevitable in the nature of medical progress, especially at the high-technology level, that full private practice could never recover a primary place in the delivery of health care. It is already priced out of most markets. Very few private practitioners can afford the supporting teams, hospitals and other services, which modern medicine demands to make it safe for patients.

Politicians tend to have grandiose schemes of bringing succour of all sorts to everybody within their jurisdictions. The resources of a country have now been shown to be incapable of doing this within the realm of health care. Something less must be the objective. This has already been argued at length in other areas of medicine. The same sort of arguments apply to private practice also. It is now peripheral to health care in advanced communities, whose concern should be to bring the health care which they can afford to as many of the people as they can. Private practice is irrelevant in this, for comparatively it takes few resources, and those that it does command are not in general available to the public health services. On the other hand, doctors should perhaps abandon the emotive arguments for the continuance of private practice by suggesting that only by direct payment of fees or insurance by the patient to the doctor is the doctor-patient relationship maintained. This is palpably untrue and casts aspersions on those doctors who elect to work full-time for some health care agency. A good doctor-patient relationship depends on the personalities of the two people involved and not on the transfer of cash. It should also depend most upon the ethos of medicine, which avowedly is that any doctor will always do the best he can for every patient in his care. This is the basis of the status of medicine, not the financial transactions that go with it.

What do the doctors want from society? What are their aspirations? The ordinary practitioners want job satisfaction, for there is a desire to be useful, otherwise they would never have started in medicine. But also they want status and a high income. At the leading edge of medicine there is also intellectual curiosity. Because many of such doctors satisfy that intellectual curiosity through research, through contact with other doctors, and through teaching, they are usually remunerated at a lower level than the other practitioners. It is odd that this is so, for it is often these more academic doctors who are preserving and advancing medicine, and it is their work which makes that of the ordinary practitioner more useful, or even alters its kind. It is, on the other hand, the intellectually curious who have had the power of persuasion and so have until recently been able to force resources into high technology and into hospitals. Their excellence has commanded support, both morally and financially, from society. Now, excellence is being called into question, as the goals of society change, and as the contribution of these leaders is beginning to be doubted medical progress is becoming the prerogative of the more ordinary. This underlies the drive for the delivery of health care in the community, under the twin guises that it is there that disease is most common and that disease caught in its early stages is preventable. Moreover, the last argument is strengthened by suggesting that such prevention will be cheaper than providing cure with high technology. All this may be spurious, for it depends upon the definition of what disease is; diagnosing diseases early does not always mean that they can be cured; and really full-blooded prevention programmes can be very costly, for they need large teams, and the result of their work is often to increase the demand for technology to deal with the cure of disease that has been unearthed.

Society seems to want from medicine maximum longevity, relief and comfort from physical and psychological distress. But it has been argued that whilst hoping for this, society does not totally will the means to achieve it, and if it were achievable the results might well be disastrous. The problem essentially is to find the form of organisation of medicine which will match the resources which society feels it can afford to give to all forms of medical activity.

The first requirement to carry out this plan is an alteration of the attitudes both within society and within medicine as to what health care is about and what it can achieve. The analysis appears to show that the aspirations and expectations, both of society and medicine, have been very unrealistic. Realism now seems to be needed. Put briefly, there needs to be acceptance that medicine is not an absolute good, but only a relative one, dependent upon what the society in which it is practised will afford. The second element in realism is getting the right time-scale. The millennium is not just round the corner for medicine, nor is it for anything else. For an enterprise as large as medicine a fairly long time-scale is needed. In Western society it takes about twelve years from the beginning of medical studies to produce a doctor of the type we have now. This consists of about six years of undergraduate study and the remainder as a postgraduate. The postgraduate years do provide some services to the community, though not perhaps as much as the doctors in those years believe.

It is often said that twelve or more years is an inordinately long time in which to produce a useful doctor. Attempts are made to reduce the length of the undergraduate curriculum and the postgraduate training. This could be done if there were acceptance of a different kind of doctor from the one we have now. It is unlikely to happen, since the whole course is controlled by the medical profession, which will not allow its standards to diminish, and because society has come to have high expectations of the expertise of its doctors. In this the public and the profession are at one, and only revolution or dictatorship would seem likely to change this attitude. If we stay with this long cycle of production of doctors and slow movement in changing the climate of opinion within society and medicine, a long planning cycle is needed. To achieve this must mean that medicine (as well as many other human, and especially intellectual, activities) has to be unhitched as far as possible from political changes. It has been emphasised that medicine cannot be removed from the political arena, for governments must have a concern for the health of their populations and also they must provide the major share of the resources, and in democracy they represent the people. But this representation is on too short a time-scale for medicine to develop rationally, in meeting the needs of society and those of the men and women who work in health care. Opposing political parties would never come to agreement on the aims and objectives of health care. The organisation of politics is such that this could not be expected. But if governments and their oppositions want the development of health care to be rational they might agree on what percentage of the gross national product they would allot to it. There might well be some other basis for agreement, but the objective must be to give medicine a firm basis on which to plan for the relatively long-term future. It must be realised too that the resources allotted may decrease as well as increase, and planning should take account of this, but there is no reason, except indulgence and impatience, why either medicine or society need spend all its available resources and assume that all expansion is needed within a short time.

If the resources can be known, within reasonable limits, then they should be handed over to an independent agency, acting on behalf of government. It could not, of course, be completely independent, since no government seems able to countenance this, but it should be given the maximum autonomy of which the political system is capable, and that autonomy should be guaranteed over a long period. This would be the trial solution advocated earlier. It implies that it may have to be changed, if experience shows it not to be working. But it needs something like a twenty-year time span before making a final assessment.

A Health Commission, set up with fair autonomy, would have the task of reconciling the legitimate interests of society with those working within health care. There can be little flexibility in the short term in doing this. Personnel take the major share of finance available, leaving only a small percentage of the budget free for change and experimentation. Experimentation here means anything new which is introduced into the service. Reverting to the Popperian philosophy, everything new is in the nature of a trial solution to a problem, and every trial solution is an experiment and not a final answer.

Such is the nature of society at present that those already working in health care have a right to expect that they will have their functions recognised, that they will be paid and that they will be given some resources with which to do their jobs. But nowadays this cannot mean that they can have the incomes that they demand, nor all the resources that they would wish. But the Health Commission would have the task of running the service, whilst agitation for increased salaries and increased resources would be directed where it should be, which is at government. It is right that government should be pressed to increase the monies they will allot to the service and even the Health Commission should do this. But it seems essential that the management of the resources available should be separated firmly from the politics of health care.

The Health Commission will need the trust of government, of the health professionals and of the public. Trust is a vital element in all human affairs and especially so in medicine, for the sick are in the hands of forces they do not understand and they are ministered to by agents whom perforce they must trust to act on their behalf. In general this trust has been built on a sound basis between society and medicine. The further building up of this trust must be a major aim, and will determine the constitution of the Health Commission.

With a Health Commission established it could take over all established health resources. There is a central core of these which is easy to define, but many others where the boundaries between health care and other services are difficult. This immediately defines tasks and problems. The task as regards the central core is to maintain the present state of affairs and keep the service going at its present level, without introducing drastic changes. In all aspects of health services, particularly the National Health Service in the United Kingdom, there has been overmuch attempt at revolution rather than evolution. A longer time-scale, which the Health Commission would give, would allow a breathing space to re-establish trust between those responsible for health care and their patients and clients. There must be a period of stability, with the immediate future not subject to sudden, often incomprehensible, vagaries. These have, in the immediate past, been the result of politics intruding too much into health care. The internal face of the Health Commission must be seen by the health workers to be as benign as possible within its allotted resources.

The external face of the Health Commission is one for definition of problems and for trial solutions. There is a whole range of social welfare, which is hard to distinguish from health services. Co-ordination of the two is often difficult, and does not necessarily respond to central legislative decree or regulation. Different solutions should be tried in different places. Another important matter of 'external' relations is that of medical education. Traditionally the undergraduate curriculum has been in the hands of the universities. There is little doubt that for the immediate future that is where it should remain. Postgraduate education and continuing education have traditionally been the sphere of the Royal Colleges. At first they were involved only in conducting examinations, but more recently they have entered the field by counselling and assisting their candidates for diplomas. Again there would seem to be no sense in trying to provide anything different at present. It is an inherited system which should be allowed to evolve. The universities too have recently been more directly concerned with postgraduate and continuing medical education. This is a very proper role, since concepts of medical education and what is required of doctors are changing rapidly. It is inevitable therefore that what is taught and learned during the undergraduate years must affect the kind of postgraduate education that is needed, and similarly the content of the postgraduate education will determine what can be left out of the undergraduate one. In general the universities and the Royal Colleges have produced the sort of doctors needed by the health services. There would appear to be no mandate for trying to find some overall solution by pushing all these activities under one umbrella. There need be nothing sacrosanct about the present system, but it does not seem to be so inordinately bad that it cannot be allowed to evolve. A major role of the Health Commission would be long-term planning, which would be possible if it was certain of what resources it could command. This would mean that better forecasts could be made of the need for doctors and other health service workers, so that there could be gradual shifts in the entry of students to their various courses, knowing the length of the cycle that is required to produce doctors and make them useful to others within the health service.

An aim of the Health Commission should be to keep out of the local decision-making processes as much as possible. It is doubtful if they should earmark grants for any purpose. There should be a willingness to trust those more close to the scene of

the action to behave responsibly. In general they will, and there
is no need for central agencies constantly to be monitoring and
expecting accounts from those in lower tiers of organisation.
To do so has been shown to be time-wasting and counter-
productive. Of course, mistakes will be made, but these should
be recognised as a price to be paid for giving authority to lower
tiers. In any case the evidence is not very substantial that central
decisions are any less likely to produce mistakes than are peripheral ones, and when the mistakes are central they are on a
grander scale and much more difficult to correct.

The reorganisation of the health service in the United Kingdom was a serious attempt to devolve responsibility as near to
the delivery of health care to individuals as possible. But it had
two defects. The first was to superimpose too many controlling
bodies over those right at the periphery of the organisation.
The second was to allow financial control of the service to
remain centralised. It is that control which breeds the mistrust.
If people are responsible enough to administer the health
services of their area, region or hospital or district, they must be
allowed to be responsible for the expenditure of money, and not
have its use determined by fiat from some more central agency.
Attitudes and practices must really change in this area of giving
authority and responsibility and in providing resources.

In monitoring what is happening in peripheral districts there
is too tight control in the present National Health Service, and a
belief that corrective action must be taken early in the development of a new scheme. This is fallacious because it means that
the corrective action is based on preconceived ideas, which may
have little justification on the evidence. 'Experiments' should
be allowed to run for some time to be sure whether they are
failing or succeeding. It is manifest to all who work peripherally
that the central agencies do not understand the details of the
local scene. Not least among these details are the differing
personalities and competences of the local people. They cannot
be legislated for. Trial solutions of local problems should be
encouraged rather than vetoed.

The Health Commission should have several Regional Com-
missions, with authority within the defined regions similar to
those of the central Commission. To avoid day-to-day inter-

ference, there should be no tier between the Regional Commission and the smaller districts where the actual delivery of health care is carried on. Block grants should be given to these peripheral areas, without special earmarking. They need autonomy, not central control; trust, not doubt. The main items of expenditure are ongoing and cannot be changed. The area of real flexibility in expenditure is minimal. But this flexibility is all-important for the health and 'experimentation' of the health services. Each tier of the organisation must keep something of its grants available for this purpose and for carrying out the Error Elimination which inevitably must follow the Trial Solutions. But the government should not be allowed to interfere directly with any of the running of the health service. It should only ever act through the Health Commission. Government is manifestly not capable of exercising managerial function in so large an enterprise as the health service, for reasons already considered. Nor does central government truly represent all the people all the time, and the same is true at local levels. Nor does democratic voting necessarily give a true picture of local needs. Those thrown up by the voting system are self-selected people with certain characteristics and ways of thought which are not shared by all. Therefore, although there is a place for local government representation on the various branches of the Health Commission, it must not be allowed to oust entirely other forms of representation. These statutory bodies must consist of professional, local government and other public representatives.

Of course, certain smaller areas of the country will lag behind others in introducing new and better schemes of health care. But this is to be expected. It has never been otherwise. Always there have been variations in facilities, resources and personnel in different regions and between countries. It is too grandiose to try to give the same health care to everyone wherever he may be. Another element of realism should be included. Moreover, there is no certainty that innovation is necessarily progress. Progress can only be judged by reference to aims. Aims are value judgements, based often in health care on inadequate grounds. Progress takes one a little closer to the aim, and regress a little further away from it. Even aims are not static, though they may be held comparatively still, if enough time is given for working towards them.

The central core of the health services is what is already present. For its proper continuance and to preserve the morale of all health workers, it is essential for the Health Commission to hold on course and give some stability, as already argued. This will be beneficial for patients too, for at least they will be able to continue with the services to which they have become accustomed. But there is the job too to be done in improving services. This means introducing better practices into areas where they are lacking, and also the encouragement of more fundamental research into the basic operations of the service, and into its science and technology. None of these can be fast, and too often the nature of the introduction of new modes of work into practice are either not thought about or are not understood.

All research begins with thinking. At a fundamental level such thought is often a flash of inspiration, an unusual juxtaposition of old ideas, rather than a logical well-thought-out hypothesis. Such a new train of thought is then tested by research into the literature and by trying it out on colleagues. It may then be realised that the idea has been worked on before, or that there is some facet of it that could do with further investigation. Rarely can this be done at a simple level nowadays, so resources have to be sought from some grant-giving body. This means that the original idea has to be judged by others who are or should be impartial, but who yet have some expertise in the particular field of investigation. This is a very difficult task. Who gets the resources, amid competing claims, depends very largely on value judgements. The quality of the idea is important, but this has to be judged against what are considered to be desirable aims and, taking two extreme examples, one body may value operational or practical research whilst another values scientific minutiae. In addition, values must be given to the quality of the researcher, the team which he may be able to command, and the resources which he already has at his disposal. Inevitably, operational research involves many others, whose co-operation is needed to gather data. They too have their own ideas and they can help or hinder according to these. In more fundamental research fewer people are involved who can interfere with the investigation. But ultimately the results of investigation have to be tried out on a wider audience. This may be by presentation at a scientific congress, or in the case of operational research it has to be introduced on a wider scale. It is here that problems come into evidence. The earlier part of the work is carried out by enthusiasts, but even they will usually agree that their results are tentative, or inconclusive and worthy of further study. There is little immediate certainty to be had in biological or psychosocial research. Inevitably, the introduction of a new idea to a larger group of people will be received with scepticism by many, with acceptance by a few and with apathy by the rest. In other words, the results of investigation have to pass the test of acceptability. But they will not be fully introduced until there is ready acceptance by a large number of those who are being asked to reduce the research to practicality. This is the aspect which is frequently ignored. And it explains why what is a self-evident advance to some is resisted.

The relevance of acceptability to the workings of the health services should be obvious. New ideas will only slowly be brought to fruition in practical terms, and they will only be brought into practice at different rates in different places. This too should occasion no surprise. But health workers will not be bludgeoned into acceptance; they can only be persuaded. Persuasion means education. This too must be a function of the Health Commission; one which has been greatly neglected in the recent past. It is vital that the Commission should be collecting information, sifting it and by education persuading its health-care workers to adopt and try out new ways of doing things. This kind of education is probably beyond its powers in the scientific and technological spheres, and must probably be left to the present methods of dissemination. The Commission will need specialists to advise it on whether a particular piece of investigation is worth introduction on a practical applied plane.

These considerations suggest that the Health Commission must keep enough of its financial resources to retain flexibility in the introduction of the results of research. It can back its persuasive powers with money, though this should be used in a positive sense and not by deliberate deprivation of a present service, which would be disruptive and destructive of morale.

The health services have four functions, which are practice, teaching, research and administration. The proposed Health Commission should leave practice, as far as possible, to those who deliver care, and give them the resources to do it, without constant central supervision. Teaching, at undergraduate and postgraduate levels in medical education, demands liaison with the universities and the Royal Colleges and other educational bodies. The universities are the primary producers of those who will be 'consumed' by the health services. Similar considerations apply to other health workers than doctors. The Health Commission must therefore be responsible for apprising the primary producers of its later needs. But it must be recognised that that depends on value judgements about the direction of medicine and what it is for and how much the community will afford for it. Medicine simply cannot continue to behave as though it were separate from the rest of society. Its role is within society and must minister to its needs, as those are felt by society. If universities, and other producers of health-care workers, decide to produce more of them than the country's health services can use, the only alternative seems to be to export these workers to countries less well endowed than themselves. At some point, therefore, it is going to be essential to determine just how many doctors, and others, will be needed. Pragmatically it has emerged that about one doctor to every 800 people will provide the sort of health service that is available now in developed countries. Perhaps the figure should be held at something like this level. Deterioration in the service would then be seen to be due to falling productivity by the doctors, in the ways already outlined. If this happened, then more doctors could be produced, but if the resources given to the Health Commission were determined then the increased number of doctors would have to share out the finances available. In other words, the doctors would have to suffer a cut in income. But it is surely no longer possible to maintain high incomes for decreasing amounts of work. There will be no income to be gained from status which is dependent upon past services, and which is not freshly earned by each generation. If status, gained through hard work and long hours and community service, which is unstinting, is discarded, it seems probable that income must diminish. As has been previously argued, those who want the high incomes will have to go to the societies which can afford them. If they do this in sufficient numbers they will depress the market for doctors' services in the recipient countries also. Only the expanding economy can keep them all in the style to which they have become accustomed, but expanding economies are becoming fewer and harder to find. Much of the trouble in medicine at the moment is due to the changes in society, in its thinking and in its values, and in its disposable resources, and medicine cannot escape any of them. When the limits are reached they affect medicine as deeply as any other activity of society.

The Royal Colleges are essentially the guardians of the conscience of medicine as well as of the minimum expertise required of those within their specialties. These too are subject to the limitations which society indirectly puts upon them. There is no point in the over-production of specialists in disciplines that are already overcrowded. They too must learn from the Health Commission what its requirements for health workers will be. And again the only alternative to holding down production will be to export medical manpower to other areas of the world. The doctors going to rich developed countries can fend for themselves. Those going elsewhere may perhaps go at the expense of the 'giving' country as a form of practical charity to the host country.

In some areas of any given country there is demonstrable maldistribution of health services, and of health workers. To remedy this requires either dictatorial powers or incentives to attract doctors. This is where the flexibility of the resources of the proposed Health Commission may be used. Various incentives might be tried, and among the most likely to be successful are those of inducement payments. When this is not possible, or will not attract, then the only alternatives are either to build up services less than those usually given by doctors, or to arrange transport of patients, by the best possible local means, to centres of health care. This could take many forms, but their kind must be dependent upon local circumstance, and so can only have trial solutions at local levels.

This analysis is not exhaustive, nor is it intended to be. It points, however, to where one form of thinking may lead and so may define trends. Always in the background are value judgements, which should be recognised for what they are. They are particularly about the aims of medicine in society. These determine then what should be done. The aims need explicit statement so that they may be rationally changed as the need arises. The time-scale is of immense importance. There is much impatience, which is made worse when politics is allowed too much weight in decisions. A method has been suggested for reducing this weight, and some of the potential problems of the Health Commission have been tentatively looked at.

Because of their powers of moral persuasion, and their key position in present advanced society, the doctors have enormous influence. They can to a great extent determine the future of medicine and its place within society. But they cannot do this by themselves as so many of them have seemed to hope. They need careful and complete analysis of the various forces which delineate their powers of action. These arise from within medicine and from within society. Medical practitioners accept the limits placed upon their powers in everyday practice, and they go along with nature where they cannot impose a different pattern upon its manifestations, in disease in their patients. They do not violently oppose nature; they work with it. When the health of the profession of medicine is in potential jeopardy it is important to go along with the forces of evolution within society and bend them to the purposes which are best for society and medicine working in concert.

Select Bibliography of Modern Studies Used in the Preparation of this Book

Barzun, Jacques, *The House of Intellect* (London, Secker & Warburg, 1959)

Cartwright, Frederick F., *Disease and History* (London, Rupert Hart-Davis, 1972)

Chardin, P. Teilhard de, *The Phenomenon of Man* (London, Collins, 1959)

Dubos, René, *The Mirage of Health* (London, George Allen & Unwin, 1960)

Eiseley, Loren, *Darwin's Century* (London, Gollancz, 1959)

Eiseley, Loren, *The Immense Journey* (London, Gollancz, 1958)

Encyclopaedia Britannica, 15th edition (1975)

Graham, Harvey, *Eternal Eve* (London, Heinemann, 1970)

Guthrie, Douglas, *A History of Medicine* (London, Nelson, 1945)

Haggard, H. W., *Devils, Drugs and Doctors* (London, Heinemann, no date)

Illich, Ivan, *Medical Nemesis* (London, Calder & Boyars, 1974)

Janssens, Paul A., *Palaeopathology: Diseases and Injuries of Prehistoric Man* (London, John Baker, 1970)

Lewin, W., 'Medicine in Society', *British Medical Journal*, **3**, 523.

Medawar, P. B., *The Uniqueness of the Individual* (London, Methuen, 1957)

Miller, Henry, *Medicine and Society* (London, Oxford University Press, 1973)

Newman, Charles, *The Evolution of Medical Education in the Nineteenth Century* (London, Oxford University Press, 1957)

Popper, Karl, *The Logic of Scientific Discovery* (London, Hutchinson, 1959)

Popper, Karl, *The Open Society and Its Enemies* (London, Routledge, 1945)

Russell, Bertrand, *The Scientific Outlook* (London, George Allen & Unwin, 1954)

Susser, M. S. and Watson, W., *Sociology in Medicine* (London, Oxford University Press, 1962)

Toulmin, Stephen and Goodfield, June, *The Architecture of Matter* (London, Hutchinson, 1962)

Toulmin, Stephen and Goodfield, June, *The Discovery of Time* (London, Hutchinson, 1965)

Toulmin, Stephen and Goodfield, June, *The Fabric of the Heavens* (London, Hutchinson, 1961)

Toulmin, Stephen, *Foresight and Understanding* (Hutchinson, 1961)

Whitehead, A. N., *Adventures of Ideas* (Cambridge, Cambridge University Press, 1943)

Whitehead, A. N., *The Aims of Education* (London, Ernest Benn, 1959)

Whitehead, A. N., *Science and the Modern World* (Cambridge, Cambridge University Press, 1943)

Willey, Basil, *The Seventeenth-century Background* (London, Penguin, 1934)